Essential Therapies, for Joint, Soft Tissue, and Disk Disorders

Robert L. Swezey

With illustrations by Mary Benz Deckert

HANLEY & BELFUS, INC.   Philadelphia

Publisher: HANLEY & BELFUS, INC.
210 South 13th Street
Philadelphia, PA 19107

Coventry University

ESSENTIAL THERAPIES FOR JOINT,
SOFT TISSUE, AND DISK DISORDERS

ISBN 0-932883-19-2

Last digit is the print number: 9 8 7 6 5 4 3 2 1

CONTENTS

PREFACE

This handbook represents a boiled-down essence of the author's more than three decades of experience in rheumatology and physical medicine & rehabilitation. It provides specific guidelines for the state of the art management of the common joint, soft tissue and discogenic disorders. These guidelines have been developed by and are in daily use at the internationally recognized Athritis & Back Pain Center at the Swezey Institute in Santa Monica, California. The therapeutic approaches to pain control, restoration of function and reconditioning have been tested in thousands of cases in a busy ambulatory rheumatological practice by the author and his physician specialist associates, in close collaboration with physical therapists, occupational therapists and patient educators, to meet the practical needs of optimal patient care. This book will provide the benefit of this knowledge and experience to you and to your patients.

Special Acknowledgments. To Mrs. Mary Benz Deckert for her outstanding illustrations in this book and for her invaluable assistance in the many illustrations used at The Arthritis & Back Pain Center and in the various books, chapters and other publications that have been derived from the work of The Arthritis & Back Pain Center.

I would also like to acknowledge and thank Peggy Hughes for her indefatigable work on the preparation of this manuscript and on so many others, and for her care and concern that the details so essential to the proper presentation of the contents of this book have not been overlooked.

Special thanks to Annette M. Swezey, M.S.P.H., for her guidance, her thoughtful criticism, her dedication to the best in patient care, and most of all for her love.

ROBERT L. SWEZEY, M.D., F.A.C.P.

DEDICATION

To The American Rheumatism Association's Council on Rehabilitative Rheumatology, whose members convinced me that this handbook was needed and that it was worth the effort and energy to write it.

INTRODUCTION

The application of rehabilitative therapies to the various categories of rheumatological disorders is a function of the diagnostic entity per se, its current impact on the musculoskeletal system of the patient, and the possibilities for preventing future impairments. In all aspects of clinical medicine, the practice of medicine is determined by an admixture of science and art. At this time in the history of medicine, exploding technologies in many areas have outstripped clinical skills, and the art (and judgment) of medicine has been shaken if not overwhelmed.

There is much less pretense of scientific dogma in the application of rehabilitative therapies. The scientific basis for many therapies remains modest and the rate of expansion of scientific knowledge is still far from exponential. Nonetheless, there are fundamental principles that have been identified with sufficient scientific substantiation to justify rehabilitative therapeutic interventions on a rational basis. Oftentimes, one must choose to apply therapies based on improving patient comfort and facilitating function, especially where adequate efficacy data are lacking, yet critical clinical observations and consensus continue to support the approach. The analogy of choosing a specific NSAID or a total knee prosthesis from the myriad options is a case in point—in both instances the basis for choice may have some scientific underpinning, but clinical experience and bias, and trial-and-error are still accepted criteria for making the therapeutic decisions.

In this book, an attempt is made to reaffirm basic principles of rehabilitative therapies and to provide an outline for their application to the more common rheumatological disorders.

GENERAL COMMENTS ON SPECIFIC DISORDERS

Some general comments about the more common rheumatological disorders follow. The reader must keep in mind the nature of the disorder in question, its severity, and its impact on the psychosocial as well as anatomical functioning of the patient. This total picture must be integrated with a detailed analysis of each region or joint that is affected, as well as with regions not affected that might be compensating in part for areas of deficient articular functioning.

Osteoarthritis is the most common disease to cause joint disorders. Although it can occur as a primary generalized disease, the selection of joints typically involves the hands symmetrically and other joints (first MTP, knee and hip) more or less at random. The various regions described in this text address these common joint problems and their rehabilitative management.

So-called **soft-tissue rheumatism** and the potpourri of tendinous, bursal, fascial, muscular, fibromyalgic and neuralgic disorders it embraces account for most of the aches and pains we must treat. These tend to be focal, although multiple areas can be affected. Each area is discussed under the appropriate regional section in the following pages of this book.

Rheumatoid arthritis (RA) is the quintessential arthritic crippler. It can ravage almost every joint and many vital organs as well. It can also be an evanescent monarticular disorder, and it can be responsible for all of the permutations and combinations in between. The clinician must first deal with the patient and the global implications of his/her disease. This demands a sensitivity to the systemic disorder, the psychosocial impact of the disease, the loss of function, and the effects of the disorder on each joint. It is not enough to treat rheumatoid arthritis as a generic medical problem, because each involved joint demands careful analysis to ascertain the extent of involvement in terms of inflammation, deformity, pain control and, above all, functional impairment.

Prophylactic measures to minimize progression of articular disease when possible must be considered. The consequences of offering what may be "preventative" therapies, via à vis overburdening the patient with a variety of tasks, treatments and devices, requires judicious analysis on a total as well as regional and joint-by-joint basis.

The nationwide interest in physical conditioning has stimulated attempts to provide aerobic exercises for arthritis. When this can be accomplished without aggravating specific joints (one must adapt activities appropriately, e.g., swimming when lower extremities are affected, and exercycle or walking when upper extremities are primarily involved), a lessening of discomfort and improved emotional status can result.[1,2,97]

We are all limited in terms of the number of pills we will swallow, the number of gadgets we will use (splints, braces, etc.), and the number of exercises or other "therapeutic activities" we will perform on a daily, let alone indefinite, basis. Failure on the part of the patient to comply with a multiplicity of therapeutic demands can add the onus of failure and guilt to the burden of the arthritic patient's suffering.

This book directs the reader to specific therapeutic options for specific joints, with the assumption that a wise and practical minimum of treatments will be employed and directed toward carefully considered goals for the whole patient and each of his or her joints.

Rheumatoid variants, including **psoriasis**, **Reiter's disease** and **colitic arthritis**, pose the same potential for joint disorders as does rheumatoid arthritis. Concern for functional positioning for joints undergoing ankylosis is a particular problem in psoriasis. **Ankylosing spondylitis (AS)** and the spinal manifestations of the rheumatoid variants pose special problems because of the predisposition to spinal deformity and involvement of axial joints with their tendency to ankylose. This is particularly true in the hips, which may remain a problem even after total joint replacement. The emphasis in treatment of ankylosing spondylitis is on maintenance of posture and mobility. This is addressed in the sections on the neck, upper back and lower back, as well as in the sections referring to the specific joints. A recently published booklet on ankylosing spondylitis details many aspects of exercise and rehabilitative therapies for the ankylosing spondylitis patient.[3]

Rehabilitation considerations for **systemic lupus erythematosus (SLE)** are complex and behaviorally oriented, dealing first and foremost with the psychological impact of a potentially life-threatening disease, drug side effects, and central nervous system involvement. Specific pain and physical disabilities are managed similarly to rheumatoid arthritis, with recognition that the joint disorder in SLE is for the most part nonerosive. Raynaud's phenomenon is discussed under the section on the hand.

Polymyositis and **steroid myopathies** can both coexist with SLE or pose problems independently. From a rehabilitative standpoint, the focus of therapy is on the activities of daily living (ADL) adaptations to facilitate movement and conserve energy. Exercise and postural emphasis designed toward maintaining joint mobility and preserving strength are the order of the day. Vigorous exercise in myopathies may cause more weakness, so activities should be designed to keep muscle function at the optimum, with exercise used to supplement functional activities.

Progressive systemic sclerosis (PSS) and "**CREST**" pose problems similar to those seen with SLE and polymyositis, and the same guidelines for therapy apply. Pulmonary compromise and the need for energy-conserving ADL techniques is a not infrequent problem in PSS. Contractures of the hands have not been demonstrated to respond well to exercise or bracing, so again ADL adaptations to enhance hand function should be given early consideration.

The rehabilitative aspects of **polymyalgia rheumatica** are either nonexistent because of the outstanding responses to steroid therapy, or the problems stem from steroid-induced myopathic and articular problems, and these are treated in the manner previously described.

For the sake of brevity, an outline format using a regional approach (e.g., Knee Disorders) has been developed and additional references for more detailed information are provided.

Principles and Aphorisms

1. PAIN CONTROL is the first consideration in any rehabilitative regimen.[98-100]
2. THE TREATMENT REGIMEN should be as brief and as simple as possible consistent with its goal (e.g., if three stretches of the shoulder one-time daily will maintain the range of motion prescribed, three one-time daily and not three three-times daily, nor 30, etc., should be prescribed).
3. ADHERENCE (compliance) to a treatment regimen at the very least requires sufficient patient instruction to achieve an understanding of its specifics and to motivate its ongoing implementation. The motivation also requires understanding the patient and his or her style, fears, beliefs and goals.
4. REST and restriction of skeletal motion can reduce inflammation but can also promote weakness and contractures. Rest must be balanced with appropriate movement whenever feasible.
5. JOINT PROTECTION PRINCIPLES:[4]
   (a) Joints protected by splints, rest, or during activities should be positioned to avoid deformities.
   (b) Transferring skills (e.g., ability to arise from a chair or get in a car) must be instructed to provide optimal independence, joint protection, safety and energy conservation.
   (c) The strongest joints should be used insofar as possible during activities (e.g., shoulder strap versus a handle on a purse).
   (d) Planning and pacing activities to minimize prolonged or excessive joint use and to conserve energy.
6. EXERCISE therapy has many objectives, and typically only one objective is achieved optimally by any specific exercise. These objectives are:
   (a) Preserve motion.
   (b) Restore lost motion.
   (c) Increase strength and static endurance.
   (d) Increase dynamic (kinetic) endurance.
   (e) Enhance a feeling of well-being.

    (f) Provide cardiovascular conditioning.

    (g) Provide active recreation.

7. SPLINTS should relieve pain or improve function, unless they are being used for specific postoperative positioning or on a temporary basis to reverse contractures.

8. THE HIERARCHY OF THERAPIES typically is:

    (a) Pain control.

    (b) Restoration of motion.

    (c) Restoration of strength.

    (d) Preservation of function.

The approach to management of rheumatological disorders must of course be based on an accurate diagnosis and medical/surgical management as well as on specific **DIAGNOSIS** of the musculoskeletal problems per se. **THERAPIES** follow logically but require specific application to the specific skeletal problem in the context of the whole patient (Table 1).

TABLE 1.   Mnemonics for Diagnosis and Therapies

D-I-A-G-N-O-S-I-S

D — **D**eformity
I — **I**nflammation
A — **A**cute-chronic
G — **G**ait abnormalities
N — **N**eurological complications
O — **O**ther medical conditions
S — **S**ites of skeletal involvement
I — **I**ntensity of pain/joint damage
S — **S**trength

T-H-E-R-A-P-I-E-S

T — **T**herapeutic modalities
H — **H**ands-on (manipulation, spray-stretch, massage)
E — **E**xercise
R — **R**est/relaxation
A — **A**DL (occupational therapy)
P — **P**sychological considerations
I — **I**mmobilization/splint/corset
E — **E**ducation
S — **S**ocioeconomic considerations

1. CERVICAL REGION

The diagnostic categories of cervical problems frequently encountered in rheumatological practice are discogenic with and without radiculopathy, rheumatoid arthritis with C1–2 involvement and/or mid- and lower cervical involvement (rheumatoid arthritis and degenerative or traumatic discogenic disease commonly co-exist), ankylosing spondylitis, and polymyositis. From the standpoint of therapies, there are certain generalizations that may apply to most of these disorders and specific issues relevant only to one or two of them. The *severity* (pain, instability, neurological deficit) and *chronicity* (acute, subacute or chronic) determine the kinds and intensities of various therapies to be applied, or indeed not applied, to any specific diagnostic category. General considerations for THERAPIES in *cervical* disorders are presented in the following, with specific comments related to specific disease entities inserted where appropriate.

CERVICAL DISORDERS

In the approach to cervical problems it is important to recognize that most discogenic and degenerative disorders of the neck affect the lower cervical spine, and then later the middle cervical spine, and relatively rarely the upper cervical spine. This pattern also is followed in ankylosing spondylitis but tends to be reversed in rheumatoid arthritis, although severe midcervical involvement can occur in the latter in the absence of C1–2 involvement and vice versa. The midcervical involvement in rheumatoid arthritis is often more subtle and sometimes more devastating than the high cervical subluxations. Ligamentous and muscular strains, and prolonged reflex muscle spasm are almost invariably present with symptomatic discogenic disorders. In any given case they may be the major pathogenic factor.

True immobilization of the C1–2 area by any brace short of the "halo" is ineffective.[5] Management of mid- and lower cervical disorders (discogenic and musculoligamentous) follows the same principles outlined below, with the reservations appropriate to the inflammatory status of rheumatoid arthritis and the restriction of cervical motion that is associated with bony fusion and inflammation in ankylosing spondylitis.

T — Therapeutic Modalities

In acute cervical pain, cold compresses used for 20 minutes on and 20 minutes off, and local ice massage to areas of local tenderness for two to three minutes prn are used for pain control. Focal *transcutaneous nerve stimulation* (TNS) (*point finder*) or regional TNS for local or radicular pain can be employed. The focal TNS or point finder can be used for periods of 30 seconds to each tender point and trigger point daily to two to three times a week, and the standard TNS can be applied for periods varying from 20 to 30 minutes up to continual use, most typically for one to two hours once or twice daily.[6–10]

Ultrasound and *superficial heat* can be offered when cold is poorly tolerated and prior to exercises.

Traction in very acute cases may not be tolerated until after a few days of immobilization. Pretesting with manual traction for tolerance and the preferred line

5

of traction force is essential. For most patients, on a home regimen, three to five minutes of 20–25 pounds of traction used twice daily with the patient seated is adequate for pain control, although 20–30 minute periods are customarily prescribed.[11,12] *Temporomandibular joint* (TMJ) problems may necessitate use of occipitofrontal head halters. In an occasional patient, special angles of pull are more comfortable (e.g., vertical rather than in mild flexion, or in 30 degrees of flexion and 30 degrees of right angulation).[13] Mechanical traction has limited value over the simpler and less expensive home traction applications—provided adequate patient instruction is given (Fig. 1).

Acupuncture (and *acupressure*) may offer an alternative pain control adjunct.[14]

In **rheumatoid arthritis** and **ankylosing spondylitis**, traction is generally poorly tolerated and not helpful. Indeed, it may lead to disastrous complications in the former if not carefully applied, and is best avoided.

FIGURE 1.   Cervical Traction.

A simple over-the-door traction apparatus is utilized. The patient is seated alongside the door in such a manner that when the tractive force is applied his head is in approximately 20° of flexion and centered so that the line of pull of traction does not deviate the head and neck from the midline. The patient, preferably in an armless chair, sits up straight and applies the halter so that when traction is applied, support is equally distributed between the chin and the occiput or is slightly greater at the occiput. He then relaxes his body and slumps in the chair and allows the weight of the upper body to serve as a traction force. This technique eliminates the need for any complex apparatus or struggling with weights. Some patients are not able to relax sufficiently to utilize this method, or the tractive force of their body weight is excessive, in which cases specific weights (7 to 15 kg) are used in the traction pulley system. Where no weight is used, the suspending rope can be either tied to the overhead pulley or attached to an adjacent doorknob. A clothesline tightener can be positioned on the rope to facilitate tension control and adjust the traction force.

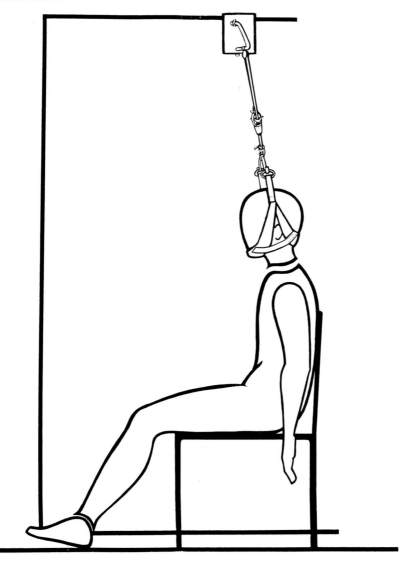

FIGURE 1. *See legend on opposite page.*

H — Hands-On

Manual traction with *slow contract-relax stretching* augmented by prior *cold spray* or *icing* is a useful modality for relieving muscle spasm and consequent restricted cervical mobility and pain. *Acupressure* over focal trigger areas can give pain relief. *Manipulation* in acute, nonradicular cervical disorders (exclusive of RA and AS) can restore pain-free mobility more rapidly than other modalities in some instances.[12,15–17] Manipulation of the cervical spine can also cause additional cervical trauma, spinal cord injury, or stroke and is best avoided in favor of active assistive or muscle energy manual therapies to increase cervical mobility, relieve pain, and restore function.[12,101]

E — Exercise

When immobilization by soft collar or brace is essential for pain control, exercises to *gently increase scapular mobility* can be initiated (Figs. 2–5). This provides a measure of relief of *general cervical and upper back stiffness* and can be followed by limited cervical range of motion exercises when tolerated (Figs. 6–11). The use of local ice or heat to relieve discomfort can facilitate exercise therapy. When cervical range of motion is improving and pain is lessened, *isometric exercises* initially applied to the neck flexors, and then to the lateral neck flexors and extensors, as well as conditioning exercises for the scapulae and upper extremities can be introduced (Fig. 12).[11] Cervical isometric strength is an important conditioning exercise prior to reduction of bracing.

Swimming with a snorkel to minimize neck motion can be well tolerated, but the breast stroke (neck hyperextends) and diving should be avoided. Bicycling in the head-up "touring" posture is recommended for those who enjoy this sport.

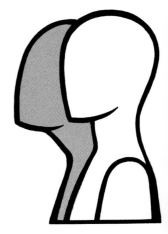

FIGURE 2. **Chin-In, Chest-Up Position.**

The purpose of this exercise is to establish head and neck alignment and a basis for head and neck positioning for neck exercises. The patient is instructed to sit with the back comfortably supported, to keep the shoulders rolled back and down, and to take a deep breath and relax while breathing out. The eyes are kept level while the chin and head move straight back. This should be associated with a sense of lengthening at the back of the neck and the head raising slightly. For some patients it is helpful to suggest that they visualize a string attached to the top of the back of their head pulling straight up to help "lengthen the neck."

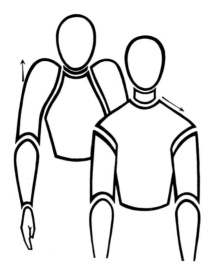

FIGURE 3. **Shoulder Shrugs with Downward Stretch.**

The purpose of this exercise is to relieve neck and shoulder tension. The patient is instructed to assume the chin-in, chest-up position, to breathe out and to relax, and then to shrug the shoulders gently up toward the ears, holding in that position for a count of three, and then relaxing the shoulders so that the fingers reach toward the floor, creating a stretch on the upper back at the base of the neck. The final position is held for a count of six, and the patient then relaxes and returns to the starting position.

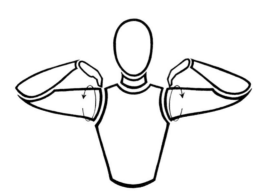

FIGURE 4. **Intermediate Shoulder Circles.**

The purpose of this exercise is to stretch and increase the range of motion in the pectorals, rhomboids, trapezii, serrati, and levator scapulae muscles. The patient assumes a chin-in, chest-up position, places his fingertips on the shoulders, and raises the elbows, pointing them away from the body by moving them directly out from the sides of the chest. The elbows are then used to draw small circles in the air about the size of a saucer, rotating first up and forward and then down and back. This is repeated until a comfortable stretch is obtained. The patient may be more comfortable wearing a soft collar, if this has been prescribed.

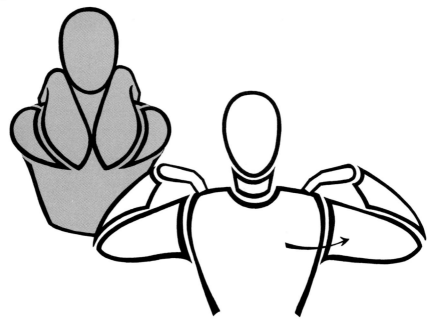

***FIGURE 5.* Elbow Touches.**

The purpose of this exercise is to stretch tense and tight muscles attached to the scapulae. The patient starts in the chin-in, chest-up position, breathing slowly in and out, and then places his fingertips on his shoulders with elbows at shoulder level. He then breathes out, bringing his elbows as close together as possible, until he gets a mild stretch in the inter-scapular area. This position is held for a count of three, and then he relaxes the arms in the start position. He then stretches the elbows behind him, bringing the scapulae close together for a stretch of the anterior chest muscles. The adducted scapular position is then held for a count of three, and the arms are returned to the start position. The exercise is repeated until a comfortable stretching has been accomplished. The patient may be able to accomplish this exercise more effectively by wearing a soft collar, if this has been prescribed.

***FIGURE 6.* Chin Tuck.**

The purpose of this exercise is to relieve neck strain by stretching the tight muscles of the back of the neck and head. This is also designed to help improve neck posture. The patient assumes a chin-in, chest-up position and places his index finger on his chin. Keeping the eyes and chin level, he moves his head gently straight back until a mild stretch is felt at the back of the neck and in the suboccipital area. He holds this stretch for a count of three to six and then resumes the start position. The exercise is repeated again three to five times until an adequate stretching has been accomplished.

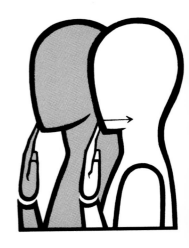

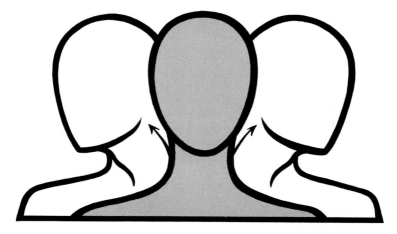

***FIGURE 7.* Beginning Neck Rotation.**

The purpose of this exercise is to restore side-to-side neck motion. The chin-in, chest-up start position is assumed, and the head is turned gently until a stretch or slight discomfort is experienced. For many patients it is easier to guide the chin to the proper position with a finger placed on the chin. The stretch position is not held and the head is returned to the start position; the same movement is then performed to the opposite side.

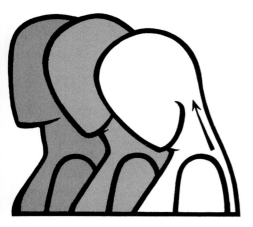

***FIGURE 8.* Forward Flexion Stretch.**

The purpose of this exercise is to loosen and stretch ligaments and muscles at the back of the neck. The patient assumes a chin-in, chest-up position, breathes in and out slowly, and then "slowly rolls" the head downward, trying to place the chin on the chest. The stretch is held for a count of three to five, and the head is then returned to the start position. This exercise can be repeated three to five times until an optimal stretch is obtained.

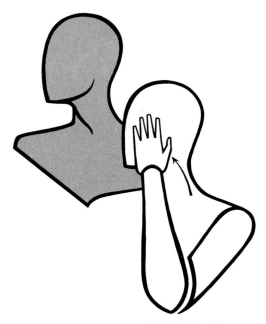

FIGURE 9.   Assisted Neck Rotation.

The purpose of this exercise is to improve neck mobility, especially when driving. The patient slowly turns the head to the right as far as possible and then takes a slow deep breath in and, while exhaling, gently pushes the head further to the right, if this can be tolerated. The head is then returned to the start position and the exercises are repeated on the opposite side. Three to five repetitions can be performed to achieve an optimal stretch.

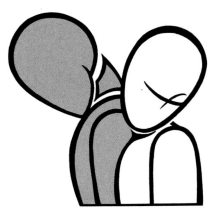

FIGURE 10.   Intermediate Neck Rotation.
(Over the Shoulder Stretch.)

The purpose of this exercise is to help restore head and neck turning motion. The patient assumes the chin-in, chest-up position and slowly rolls his head downward, trying to place the chin on the chest. This should create a stretch at the back of the neck from the weight of the head hanging as though it were unsupported. The chin is then kept as close to the chest as possible and the head rotated first to the right in an attempt to stretch sufficiently to see over the right shoulder. When the optimum stretch is achieved it should be held for 3 to 5 seconds. The process is then repeated on the opposite side.

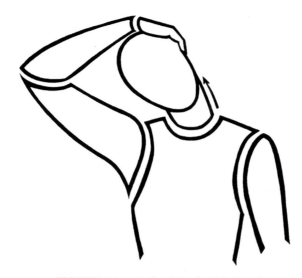

FIGURE 11. **Assisted Neck Side Bend.**

The purpose of this exercise is to improve lateral mobility of the neck. The patient assumes the chin-in, chest-up position, breathes in and out, and while exhaling bends the right ear toward the right shoulder. The right hand is then placed on the left side of the head and this further assists the stretch of the head toward the right ear. The stretch is held for a count of six. The patient then is instructed to relax, to resume the start position, and to repeat the exercise on the opposite side.

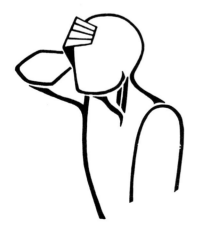

FIGURE 12. **Neck Flexor Strengthening.**
(Manually Resisted Isometric.)

The hand is placed on the forehead and resists contraction by the neck flexors. The neck extensors, lateral flexors, and rotators can be similarly exercised with the hand placed to offer resistance appropriately. Each contraction is held for six seconds, and the exercise is performed once to twice daily.

R — Rest

Rest with a *pillow* thick enough to produce support to the head in a side-lying position and thin enough to allow supine head positioning without flexion is usually most comfortable in cervical disorders. In **ankylosing spondylitis** a pillow is best avoided; however, where some flexion contracture has already occurred, a small pillow to support the back of the head in the supine posture or folded to support the side of the head in the side-lying position is helpful. A variety of pillows recommended for neck posture are available. In general, they give gentle support to the back of the neck when supine and are thickened to minimize lateral neck flexion when side-lying. A trial-and-error basis for pillow selection (like NSAIDs) is the only way to determine efficacy in any given patient. Rest while seated or driving requires *good back support* (Fig. 13), and for reading or watching television or using a computer, optimal lighting and properly refracted glasses are essential. A tilted desk or desktop slant-board at a 15 to 20 degree slope and alignment of *head and eye* to objects (CRT, book, documents) are stressed.

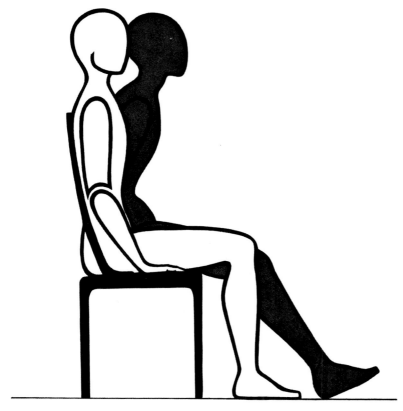

FIGURE 13. Posture, Sitting.

For proper alignment in the seated posture, the placement of the head is such that the external auditory meatus is on a plumb line that extends laterally through the shoulder and the greater trochanter. In a standing posture this line is extended to pass on the anterior lateral surface of the knee and to terminate (with the foot flat on the floor) on a point just anterior to the ankle. When seated the spine should be supported by the back rest, and this is facilitated by allowing ample space for the buttocks to protrude posteriorly or to be supported by an appropriately shaped and cushioned back support. The thighs are horizontal or in approximately 95° of flexion, the knees in 90° of flexion, and the feet are planted (with the ankles at 90°) firmly on the floor or on a stool. There should be approximately the width of a fist between the popliteal space and the sloped and preferably padded surface of the anterior of the chair to minimize pressure on popliteal neurovascular structures. There should be room between the chair legs so that the feet can be placed beneath the chair to facilitate transfer to the standing position. Alternatively, one or both feet may be placed on a low stool or on a strut fitted between the rockers of a rocking chair. The exact seating alignment will depend on the activities engaged in while sitting, and they may range from slight reclining for relaxation, television viewing, and relaxed reading to the vertical position, shown above for desk work or eating. The contrasted figure is illustrated in a slumped posture that creates hyperextension and stress on the neck and hyperflexion and stress on the lumbosacral junction.

A — ADL

Postural considerations as outlined above emphasizing the chin-in position (Fig. 2) must be reinforced. Long flexible straws and special cups and glasses facilitate *drinking* for patients in a brace or with cervical rigidity, and *prism glasses* under similar circumstances for reading in bed are helpful. Arrangement of the home and work place with objects in easy reach, preferably at or near eye level, is taught. A *hands-off telephone* or avoiding cradling the telephone is extremely important in home and work activities. In *driving*, the wide-angle rear-vision mirror, particularly for patients who must drive with a neck brace or with rigid cervical spine, is an essential safety feature. *Reacher sticks* and *footstools* for reaching up or getting under, and *instruction* for proper doffing and donning of *clothing* and *braces* must be given so as to avoid neck strain.

P — Psychological Problems

Psychological counseling as needed for chronic pain, disability, sexual dysfunction and psychopathology should be provided. Hypnosis and guided imagery training can be useful for intractable pain problems.[99]

I — Immobilization

The hierarchy of immobilization begins with a *soft collar* designed to position the head in slight flexion and to limit extension.[5] This is usually helpful in all disorders as a pain-control measure and can be worn day and night as needed. When *more rigid support* is required, as in discogenic disease with **cervical radiculopathy**, a *Philadelphia collar* (Fig. 14) carefully fitted will almost always provide sufficient immobilization to permit pain control and stabilization of neurological deficits.[5,11] Rarely a *SOMI brace* (Sub-Occipito-Mental Immobilizer) (Fig. 15) with a firm chest fixation is required for pain and/or neurological control.[5] The "halo" is required in cases with severe cervical instability and neurological deficits as occurs rarely in **rheumatoid arthritis**.[5] **Polymyositis** patients will sometimes require a soft collar or a Philadelphia collar to support the head, but care is necessary in the presence of severe cervical weakness to see that prolonged chin pressure does not lead to maceration and ulceration.

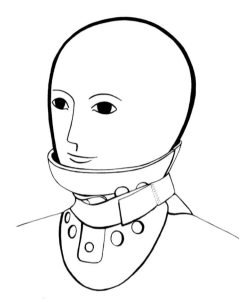

FIGURE 14. Philadelphia Cervical Brace.

This is a plastic, commercially available brace that is readily adjustable and comfortable to wear. It provides good stabilization of the entire spine and is especially effective for stabilizing the lower cervical vertebrae. It should be positioned to hold the head in slight flexion with close coaptation of occipital, submental, dorsal and sternal contacts. It is useful in moderate to severe cervical problems that do not require absolute immobilization. It serves as a comfortable alternative to the slightly more efficient immobilizing but more uncomfortable SOMI brace (Fig. 15). The chief disadvantage of the Philadelphia brace is that it tends to be uncomfortable in warm weather. For most cervical problems in which severe subluxations and/or neurological complications have not occurred, the use of a soft felt or foam rubber padded collar, or a plastic or plastic and metal collar, designed without specific suboccipital, submental, or chest contact points, will usually provide sufficient stabilization to provide pain relief.

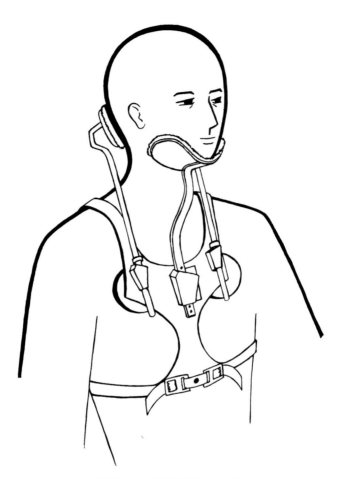

FIGURE 15.   SOMI Cervical Brace.

   A plastic and metal rigid brace that requires careful adjustment and fitting. Firm sub-occipital and submental supporting plates are rigidly held by a removable bar to a chest plate. The chest plate is held firmly to the chest by over-the-shoulder and under-the-arm straps. This brace provides excellent stabilization of the lower cervical spine and is comparable to the ''fourposter'' and Philadelphia braces in stabilization of the middle and upper cervical areas. It tends to be uncomfortable and is particularly difficult to wear when lying down. It is useful for the patient with mild radicular deficits that do not require absolute cervical stabilization. S O M I — SubOccipital Mental Immobilizer.

E — Education

The disease entity, its implications for cervical spine involvement, and methods of control must be taught. The use of any equipment (TNS, pillows, traction) and neck protective doffing and donning techniques for clothes and braces, as well as the exercise regimen, must be carefully explained and then accurately demonstrated to the patient. Adherence to any regimen requires an understanding of that regimen as well as the ability to perform it, if success in compliance is to be achieved.

S — Socioeconomic

Socioeconomic issues must be raised with each patient, and assistance in problem solving should be provided for home, work and recreation.

2. SHOULDER DISORDERS

Shoulder disorders most often involve the soft tissue structures (tendons or bursae) and are often attributable to overuse or shoulder-outlet impingement dysfunctions. These disorders can range from mild pain on specific movements to severe incapacitating pain, stiffness and loss of motion. The former are typically associated with focal tenderness in the biceps groove or rotator tendon insertions, and the latter with any of the above areas of focal tenderness and/or diffuse tenderness around the glenohumeral joint, (adhesive capsulitis or shoulder-hand syndrome). In rheumatoid arthritis, there is typically tenderness over the anterior joint capsule and varying degrees of swelling, restriction of motion, and glenohumeral subluxation due to capsular arthritis and articular resorption. These findings can be seen in ankylosing spondylitis and systemic lupus erythematosus as well as other rheumatoid variant conditions. In the case of systemic lupus erythematosus, the shoulder may be affected by aseptic necrosis, and this not uncommonly necessitates a total shoulder arthroplasty for pain control and functional restoration.

The acromioclavicular joint tends to fuse in ankylosing spondylitis and is commonly affected by osteoarthritis either spontaneously or as a result of prior acromioclavicular separations. Osteoarthritis affecting the glenohumeral joint, however, is relatively rare except as a secondary event (post-traumatic, post-RA, or associated with chondrocalcinosis).

Shoulder disorders are also common concomitants of cervical conditions by virtue of referred pain and/or overt radiculopathies. It is not uncommon for patient to suffer a chronic "**whiplash**" cervical flexion-extension injury and, while still wearing a neck brace and engaging in sedentary activities, to develop manifestations simulating an "overuse" syndrome of the rotary cuff or biceps tendon or "a tennis elbow." The cervical disorder obviously must be treated, but the shoulder requires local therapy for pain control and restoration of function, even though pathogenetically it is manifesting local pathology secondary to a primary cervical focus. Reflex *"trigger" areas* distal to the glenohumeral joint per se are commonly seen with cervical-referred as well as primary shoulder or periarticular shoulder disorders and can be found in the pectoralis major muscle (lateral border), the deltoid insertion on the humerous, and in the origin, belly, and insertions of the teres minor with great frequency.

Acute severe shoulder pain is typically crystal-induced (calcific rotator cuff tendinitis-bursitis, or gout or pseudogout). Rarely sepsis will be etiologic. **Shoulder pain with true weakness** (not painful inhibition of strength) suggests cervical radiculopathy or a rotator cuff tear. "Conservative" treatment of the latter can include surgical repair.

In all shoulder problems the priorities of treatment are pain control and restoration of mobility as soon as exercises can be tolerated.[102] Strengthening should only be initiated if pain is absent at rest and when only mild pain is provoked at the extremes of available shoulder motion.

SHOULDER DISORDERS

T — Therapeutic Modalities

The application of heat, cold and TNS is as described under **Cervical Disorders**. Shoulder abduction-external rotation-flexion *traction* in the treatment of **adhesive capsulitis** has been successfully employed for one to two hours daily in conjunction with TNS for pain control.[18]

H — Hands-On

"Acupressure" or a steady, slightly undulating, deep, firm index-finger pressure held for about 7 seconds over tender points and trigger points can be used in the clinic and by the patient at home as well for pain relief.[12,14]

Deep transverse friction massage (the index and/or middle fingertips are pressed against the bony surface of a tender biceps groove or rotator cuff insertion and a slow, firm motion of the fingertips across the longitudinal direction of the tendon fibers is applied without removing the finger contact with the bone surface) can be repeated two to three times per week until pain relief is achieved.[12,15–17]

Manual traction with *mobilization* in a graded fashion to the scapular, costal and glenohumeral areas is useful for pain control in noninflammatory shoulder problems, and it also can provide assistance in restoration of motion.[16,17]

Slow "*contract–relax*" or "*muscle energy*" mobilization techniques and *spray-and-stretch* techniques can facilitate pain control and relaxation of muscle spasms during these stretching procedures (Fig. 16A,B,C).[19–21] In occasional refractory cases where pain and restriction of motion interfere with useful function, mobilization under anesthesia is an option.

FIGURE 16A, B, C. Rhythmic Stabilization.
(Manually Assisted Manipulation.)

This is basically a passive stretching method, shown here as it is applied to the shoulder. The forearm is positioned in the extreme of its comfortable range and then a series of alternating strong isometric contractions of abductors and/or external rotators followed by adductors and internal rotators is made. Each contraction is held for about three seconds and the series of contractions consists of two or three cycles of alternating agonist and antagonist contractions. The muscle relaxation that follows the period of contractions is usually sufficient to permit the "manipulator" to passively move the joint beyond the previous limit. This process is then repeated until the maximum range for the session is attained. Rhythmic stabilization sessions can be performed daily and used as a supplement to other shoulder-mobilizing exercises, and may be effectively repeated as infrequently as weekly until a plateau of maximum range of motion is achieved. This same method can be employed in patients with painful muscle spasm limiting cervical motion.

In Figure 16A, alternating resistance to internal rotation and extension of the shoulder is shown.

In Figure 16B, alternating resistance to the external rotators and abductors of the shoulder is shown. In actuality the arm is placed in the position of maximum tolerated external rotation and abduction with resistance initially applied to the internal rotators and/or extensors, as this is the direction of least discomfort. This contraction is then cycled with a contraction in the same position of the external rotators and/or abductors and then alternated again with the internal rotators, as described above.

Figure 16C shows the relaxed shoulder (post-rhythmic stabilization) passively stretched or lifted to the newly tolerated range of motion.

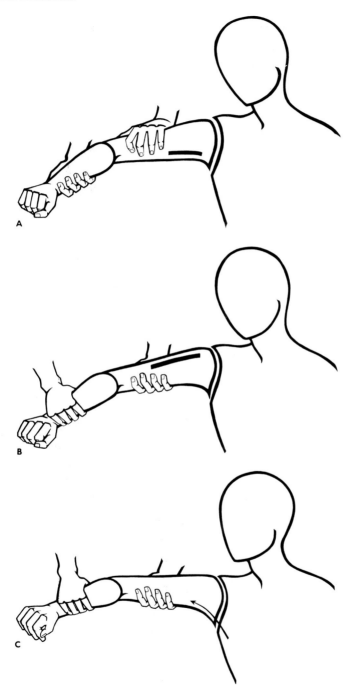

FIGURE 16.   *See legend on opposite page.*

E — Exercises

Stretching. In **acute severe shoulder disorders**, even passive motion may not be tolerated, e.g., acute calcific bursitis. Early movement can be initiated by scapular stretches without causing pain in the glenohumeral joints. The *Codman's gravity-assisted pendulum exercise* (Fig. 17) is an excellent beginning range of motion maneuver, and this can be followed as pain is controlled by "*wand-*" (golf putter, tennis racket, broom handle, cane, etc.) assisted or towel-assisted stretches into flexion external rotation and internal rotation as required and as tolerated (Figs. 18–20).[11] Horizontal abduction and adduction can then be added, but vertical abduction that impinges the greater tuberosity of the humerus against the acromion is best left for last—and if all of the other planes are well stretched, this usually proves unnecessary. Reciprocal pulleys (Fig. 21) are rarely needed in rheumatological disorders, but "*wall walking*" (Fig. 22) and doorway stretches can be effectively used in chronic mild cases of **adhesive capsulitis**.[11]

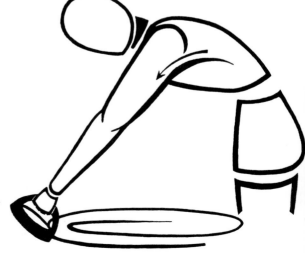

FIGURE 17. Gravity-Assisted Pendulum Stretching. (Codman Exercise.)
The patient bends forward and gravity assists the shoulder and arm in a rotary and/or pendulum motion to stretch into flexion, extension, and abduction. This can be performed with a patient standing or lying prone over the edge of a bed. In the standing position the exercise is best performed with the patient supporting himself by leaning on a table top or chair.

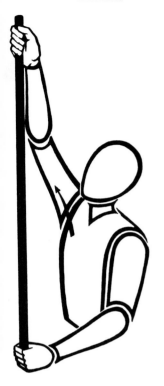

FIGURE 18.   Wand-Assisted Exercise #1. (Stretching.)

A stick, cane, baton, or wand is held in the unaffected hand, which assists ranging of the affected shoulder by pushing or pulling in the desired direction. Forward flexion is illustrated above. With the wand (or a towel) placed behind the back, external rotation or internal rotation can be performed (see Fig. 20). This exercise can be employed in the presence of moderately active inflammation of the shoulder and is particularly useful when efforts are being made to restore mobility at a time when inflammation has largely subsided.

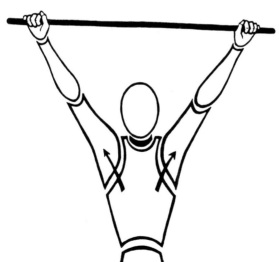

FIGURE 19.   Wand-Assisted Exercise #2. (Stretching.)

In this exercise the wand in the unaffected hand assists in a bilateral stretching movement. This exercise is enhanced by visual monitoring when performed in front of a mirror.

***FIGURE 20.*   Shoulder Internal
Rotation Stretch.**

The purpose of this exercise is to
maintain or improve internal rotation of
the shoulder. The patient can stand or
sit on a stool. A stick or towel is placed
in the right hand and then grasped from
below with the left hand, and the right
hand gently pulls the left arm up toward
the interscapular area until a comfortable stretch is achieved. The hand is
held in this position for a count of three
and then the stretch can be repeated three
to five times, and then performed on the
opposite side if indicated.

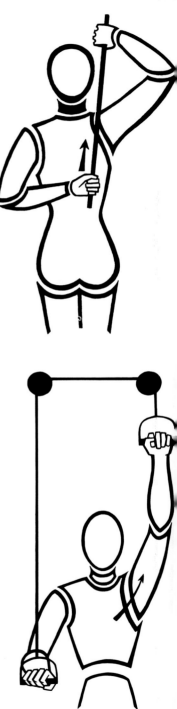

***FIGURE 21.*   Reciprocal Pulley.
(Pulley-Assisted Stretching.)**

The ''good'' arm pulls down on
one end of the pulley system and assists
the affected arm in stretching. Changing
the patient's position under the pulley
system permits assisted stretching in the
various planes of motion.

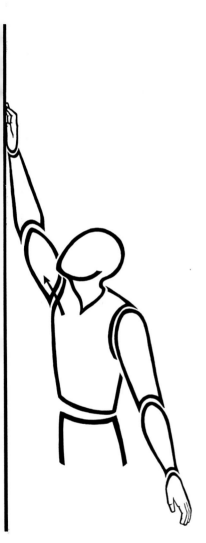

FIGURE 22. **"Wall Walking."**
(Friction-Assisted [Wall]
Stretching.)
Friction between the fingers and the wall assists in actively stretching the shoulder. A mark placed at the highest attained stretch provides a guide to progress. Flexion and abduction are effectively stretched by facing the wall and standing parallel to it, respectively.

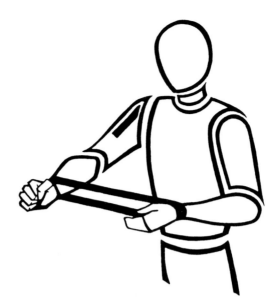

FIGURE 23.   **Shoulder Deltoid—External Rotator Strengthening.**
(Belt-Resisted Isometric.)
    The elastic band or belt is looped over both wrists. Abduction and external rotation of
the right shoulder is resisted by the opposite arm. The maximum contraction is held for 6
seconds and the exercise is performed once or twice daily.

    Strengthening.   Strengthening exercises are progressed from deltoid *isomet-
ric* exercises, performed with the forearm in a relatively adducted position (against
the chest) to minimize motion of the shoulder (using heavy dental dam, bungee,
beach ball, bathrobe sash, or pillow for resistance). Subsequently, wrist-restricted
isometrics in internal and external rotation (Fig. 23) and then biceps and triceps
resisted isometrics (Fig. 24) can be added to the shoulder-strengthening regimen.
When these can be handled without discomfort, *low resistance isokinetics* or free
weights can be progressively added until the desired goal is reached, when appropriate specific sport conditioning with proper warm-ups and cool-downs commences.[11]

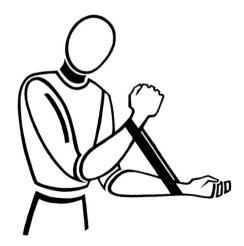

FIGURE 24. **Biceps-Triceps Strengthening.**
(Belt-Resisted Isometric.)

The right biceps and left triceps in this illustration are opposed in an isometric contraction resisted by an elastic band or belt. The elasticity is such that at the maximum contraction no motion is possible and the tension of the elastic band provides proprioceptive stimulation to encourage a maximally forceful contraction for isometric strengthening. The contraction is held for 6 seconds.

R — Rest

Avoidance of unnecessary movement or activity that might exacerbate pain and/or inflammation in the shoulder.

A — ADL

Patient should be taught pacing to avoid overuse of the shoulders, using two hands rather than straining one. Work areas should be organized, with closets, tools, and kitchen storage modified to minimize reaching. Use "reachers," step stools or ladders when necessary. Use shopping carts and carry small rather than large packages. Use "airline luggage caddys" when possible for carrying briefcases and heavy objects around town as well as when traveling.[4,22,23]

P — Psychological Problems

Counseling for chronic pain management and *hypnosis* (and/or guided imagery) can be helpful in managing refractory chronic pain problems.

I — Immobilization

Use of *slings* for support of acute-severe painful shoulders and on occasion (e.g., when traveling or in crowds) in some subacute moderate-severe cases.

E — Education

Apply basic principles.

S — Socioeconomic

Apply basic principles.

3. ELBOW DISORDERS

Two of the most common elbow problems seen by rheumatologists and physiatrists are lateral and medial **epicondylitis**.[103] Almost as common as lateral epicondylitis is referred cervical pain to the lateral epicondylar area and forearm extensor motor point (located about an inch and a half distal to the lateral epicondyle on the radial dorsal aspect of the forearm). A common concomitant of this pain-referral pattern is a tender trigger area in the supinator muscle (palpable in the distal antecubital space overlying the head and proximal shaft of the radius), which can be associated with slight restriction of elbow extension and supination.[19] Enthesitis of the forearm extensor aponeurosis laterally and the forearm flexor aponeurosis medially at the attachments to the epicondyles often responds well to local transverse *friction massage* for two to five minutes twice weekly.[16] *Ultrasound* and particularly local steroid injections are useful. The trigger point in the region of the forearm extensor motor point and the supinator muscle trigger areas typically respond well to *ice massage* and/or *spray-and-stretch*, and occasionally require local lidocaine injection to obtain relief.[19]

Rheumatoid arthritis commonly affects the elbow joint, causing pain, heat, swelling and restriction of elbow motion. This can progress to severe joint destruction. Preservation of a functional range of elbow motion in flexion is crucial for eating and grooming. **Olecranon bursal swelling with nodules** in rheumatoid arthritis and **tophi** in gout are not uncommon. Bursal drainage must be done with particular care to prevent infecting these vulnerable tissues. Local steroid (2–5 mg of triamcinolone) injections into rheumatoid nodules can appreciably reduce their size, minimize pressure-related discomfort, and improve cosmesis.[24]

T — Therapeutic Modalities

Ice as cold packs for acute inflammation, trauma, after vigorous exercise, or as *ice massage* for two to three minutes four times daily and prn to trigger areas is a useful pain control modality. *Ultrasound* (and/or friction massage) can help relieve symptoms of subacute and chronic epicondylitis. Hot soaks or compresses can be used for comfort and prior to stretching exercises in **rheumatoid arthritis**. *Spray-and-stretch* techniques may facilitate stretching of the supinator and forearm extensor muscle triggers.[19]

H — Hands-On

Friction massage to subacute and chronic moderate to severely painful epicondylar areas two to three times a week for two to five minutes is a useful pain control measure.[13] Wrist manipulation by rapid extension of the elbow with the wrist held in hyperflexion is a traditional manipulation to stretch adhesions in the extensor aponeurosis for chronic lateral epicondylitis.[16] *Acupressure* massage over trigger areas and/or *spray-and-stretch* techniques applied to the supinator and the forearm extensors may be useful in alleviating discomfort associated with lateral epicondylitis.

E — Exercise

Stretching. Forcible exercise to stretch elbow contractures (with the exception of the tennis elbow manipulation) are best avoided because of the risk of articular damage. Gentle, active assisted range of motion in flexion, extension, pronation, and supination is indicated for the arthritic elbow (Fig. 25).[11]

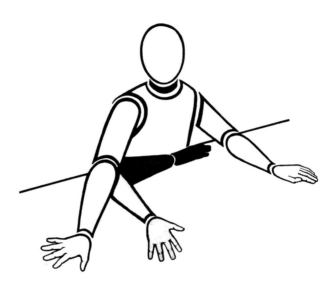

FIGURE 25. Elbow Flexion-Extension Stretching.
(Friction-Assisted [Desk Top] Gravity Eliminated [Horizontal Position])
The forearm is placed on a desk top for support. The elbow is flexed and extended, utilizing the support of the table as well as the friction of the table to assist in stretching.

Strengthening. When painfree movement has been restored (full range of motion in epicondylitis) and a range of motion adequate for light functional activities in RA (e.g., eating), then strengthening by *isometric exercise* should be commenced. Manual resistance is applied to the dorsum of the hand and then into the palm as forcefully as possible for approximately six seconds, and this can be repeated twice (two repetitions equal one set) twice daily (Fig. 26).[11] Resistance can also be supplied with heavy dental dam, bungee, beach ball, etc. (Fig. 27). The force that is used should be capable of resisting all movement until more stressful isotonic exercise can be tolerated (Fig. 28). When these isometric exercises can be accomplished without aggravating pain (usually after two to four weeks), *isotonic exercises* with light weights can be commenced and progressed until full functional activities can be performed without pain. At that time, athletics such as golf or tennis can usually be successfully commenced.

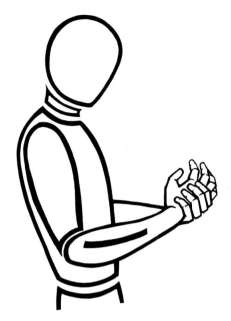

FIGURE 26.   Wrist Extensor Strengthening.
(Manually Resisted Isometric Contraction of Wrist Extensors.)
The patient uses one hand placed over the dorsum of the other hand to resist extension during a maximum isometric contraction of 6 seconds' duration.

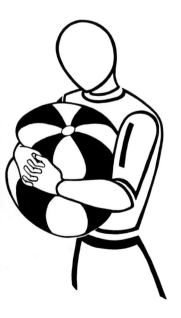

FIGURE 27.   Biceps Strengthening.
(Beach Ball-Resisted Isometric.)
A partially inflated beach ball is forcibly squeezed until no further movement is possible, and the isometric contraction is held for 6 seconds. The compression of air within the beach ball yields until it offers maximal resistance. The compression gives proprioceptive feedback to reinforce the strength of the muscle contraction. The exercise is performed for 6 seconds at maximal compression. The beach ball can be placed in various positions to exercise different muscle groups, e.g., between the lateral thigh and a wall for isometric hip abductor strengthening.

FIGURE 28. **Elbow-Wrist Pronation-Supination Stretching. (Active-Assisted with a Stick or Light-Weight Hammer.)**

The wrist and elbow are pronated and supinated as the stick is rotated. Shoulder motion is eliminated by the position of the forearm adjacent to the chest wall.

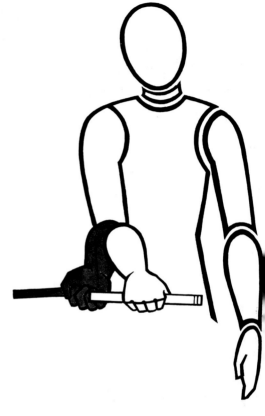

R — Rest

(See Immobilization.)

A — ADL

Modify activities of daily living for elbow protection. If the dominant side is affected, encourage the use of two hands or nondominant usage (e.g., offer the left hand for a handshake).

P — Psychosocial

Pain and/or frustration due to disability, if persistent, may necessitate counseling.

I — Immobilization

In an acute severe lateral **epicondylitis**, a forearm *cock-up splint* (readily available from surgical equipment suppliers) can be used to relieve the stretch on the forearm extensor muscles.[11] This problem may be sufficiently severe to require the additional use of a *sling*. As epicondylitis subsides, a *forearm elastic "tennis elbow strap"* worn snugly about two inches distal to the epicondyles helps unload the strain on the muscle attachments. This can be worn all day until pain is controlled and then only during vigorous activity (e.g., tennis, golf, carpentry).

In **rheumatoid arthritis**, a plastic half-open elbow splint or *"gutter"* *splint* bent to permit optimal hand function (e.g., 90 degrees for writing) can be used for support and partial elbow immobilization.

E — Education
Apply basic principles.

S — Socioeconomic
Apply basic principles.

4. WRIST AND HAND DISORDERS

The wrist and hand problems for the clinician go hand in glove (so to speak) and will be considered together because wrist problems always impact on hand function. One of the most common wrist problems is a **ganglion**. If symptomatic, local steroid injections will usually cause subsidance for prolonged periods (Bible smashing of ganglions is no longer popular). Surgical excision of ganglions does not guarantee against recurrence.[104]

Radiographic **chondrocalcinosis** of the triangular cartilage is quite common, but symptomatic pseudogout, or gout for that matter, in the wrist is not.

Rheumatoid arthritis and **rheumatoid variants** often affect the wrist with various manifestations ranging from bland dorsal extensor tendon sheath swelling to painful tenosynovitis and/or tendon rupture (particularly common in the finger extensors) and to severe destructive carpal arthritic subluxations, contractures or bony fusions.

Osteoarthritis of the first CMC joint is the most common clinical problem.

The **carpal tunnel syndrome**, which is most often idiopathic, can be associated with any of the above entities as well as a number of metabolic disorders (e.g., myxedema, pregnancy, amyloidosis). Hand pain, typically more intense in the thumb and/or index finger and often associated with numbness, tingling and weakness, may have its origins in the carpal tunnel. Like all rheumatological conditions, treatment of the local condition must be accompanied by appropriate management of any associated underlying systemic disorder and vice versa.

Common to all wrist and hand disorders is the need to reduce wrist strain (when the wrist is involved) by modification of activities of daily living and/or splinting the wrist in a manner that restricts wrist motion yet permits the maximum possible hand function.

The *thumb*, essential for dexterity and forceful grasp, is subject to a variety of disorders. Median nerve compression of the carpal tunnel typically affects the thumb and index finger. **de Quervain's stenosing tenosynovitis** of the long thumb extensor is experienced in the thumb, with tenderness over the lateral aspect of the radial styloid a frequent accompaniment. The anatomic snuffbox at the end of the base of the thumb (the first CMC joint) is the locus of most **osteoarthritis** affecting the thumb, although the first MCP and IP joints are both commonly affected. A *simple splint* (Fig. 29) modified to restrict more CMC or MCP motion, depending on the locus of involvement, serves to permit useful thumb function while protecting against excessive strain in de Quervain's disease, as well as in osteoarthritis of the first CMC and MCP joints.[11,17]

The thumb IP and MCP joints can be affected by both osteoarthritis and rheumatoid arthritis. An elastic, plastic or metal IP joint splint (Fig. 30) can provide stability to these joints. A moderately restrictive elastic sleeve splint can be used to restrict excessive movement and irritation of the tendon sheath in flexor tenosynovitis of the thumb or fingers (Fig. 31).[11]

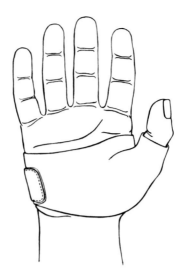

FIGURE 29. **Thumb CMC-MCP Stabilizing Splint, Plastic.**

This is a thermo-labile plastic custom-molded splint designed to provide moderate restriction of the CMC and MCP joints of the thumb. It allows for full IP flexion in order to permit optimal thumb function. The distal palmar edge of the splint is proximal to the distal palmar crease so as not to restrict MCP motion in the fingers. This splint is useful in CMC and MCP arthritis of the thumb and in de Quervain's disease.

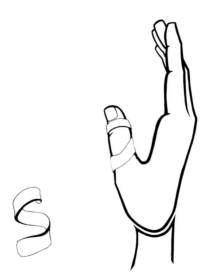

FIGURE 30. **Thumb IP Stabilizing Splint.**

The splint is metal and designed as a coil. The palmar coil lies just proximal to the IP joint, allowing for flexion of that joint, while the two dorsal surfaces of the coil resist IP extension. There is maximal thumb skin surface exposed to facilitate sensation and function. The splint can be fabricated out of plastic but when a thermo-labile plastic material is used it cannot be worn during exposure to warm surfaces or hot water.

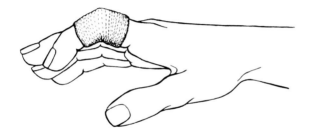

FIGURE 31. Trigger Finger PIP Splint, Elastic.

This is a 1-inch-wide elastic band sewn to make a snug (not tight) sleeve overlying the PIP joint of a finger. The elasticity permits flexion of the PIP joint from zero (extension) to about 60 to 70° of flexion. This mild restriction of PIP flexion is compatible with most functions but restricts the full excursion of the flexor tendons and thereby minimizes tenosynovial irritation and "triggering."

The **hand** can be involved joint by joint and tendon by tendon in **rheumatoid arthritis**, **variant disease** and **systemic lupus erythematosus**. Each articular structure requires specific consideration, and treatment of all structures must be assessed in the context of minimizing pain while making available and preserving optimal function. Selective local steroid injections can play an important role in conjunction with other rehabilitative therapies in suppressing local symptomatology.

The temptation to over-treat by *over-splinting* and over-exercising joints of the hands is understandable but deplorable—until and unless efficacy of the splints or exercise (other than as demonstrated by patient comfort and improved function) can be established in controlled studies. This dictum specifically applies to attempts to prevent ulnar deviation or boutonniere and swan-neck deformities by splinting. Again, if function is improved and pain ameliorated, the efforts are worthwhile but otherwise best avoided outside of a prospective study protocol.

Raynaud's phenomenon should be prevented if possible by avoidance of chilling and of smoking, and by the use of protective gloves. Skin temperature warming with biofeedback can reduce the number and intensity of ischemic episodes.[25]

Prevention of contractures in **progressive systemic sclerosis** thus far seems refractory to efforts to achieve this objective by means of splinting and exercise.[26] Whether or not **Dupuytren's contractures** are modified by any local therapy or exercise is moot—but it is hard to resist the temptation to advise gentle stretching to attempt to minimize deforming contractures for both PSS and Dupuytren's contractures.

T — Therapeutic Modalities

The specificity of various forms of heat or cold and TNS in hand problems is not great. *Paraffin* is a time-honored superficial heating modality but only an occasional patient feels it is worth the bother. Cold in particular is avoided with Raynaud's phenomenon and other cold sensitivity disorders.

H — Hands-On

With the possible exception of mobilization of a postsurgical or post-traumatic MCP or PIP contracture, there is little occasion for manual therapies for the hand and wrist in rheumatological disorders.

E — Exercises

Stretching. Active assisted range of motion to help prevent wrist contractures should be considered for flexion, extension, pronation and supination. Similar stretches seem appropriate, although unproven, when used to minimize thumb adduction contractures, to maintain intrinsic length in impending swan-neck deformities, and to maintain PIP and DIP extension in boutonniere deformities or with Heberden's nodes (Figs. 32–36).

Radial deviating stretches for ulnar deviation deformities in rheumatoid arthritis are of no known value and, although they may seem reasonable on an empirical basis, it also seems unreasonable to demand that patients perform them.[11] Assisted wrist stretching can maintain or restore range of motion (Fig. 37).

Strengthening. The benefits of strengthening exercise for various hand and wrist disorders (other than postoperatively) have not been established and indeed may aggravate deformities. *Ball squeezing is rarely justified* in an arthritic hand. Hand strength improves through usage as pain is controlled (e.g., grip strength improvement in RA), and supplementary exercises to increase hand strength in the presence of inflammation or deformity have not demonstrated any additional benefit.

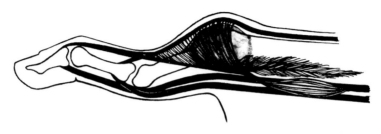

FIGURE 32. Intrinsic Muscle Anatomy.
Contractures of the interosseous and lumbrical muscles as a consequence of metacarpophalangeal (MCP) joint inflammation create tension on the finger extensor tendon mechanism. The result is MCP flexion and proximal interphalangeal (PIP) hyperextension. Elasticity of the large flexor digitorum profundus muscle creates traction on the distal interphalangeal (DIP) joint. The result is a swan neck deformity.

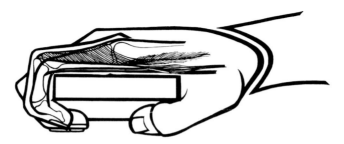

**FIGURE 33. Bunnell Exercise—DIP and PIP Flexion with
Stretching of Intrinsic Musculature.**
The lengthening of the long finger extensor tendons that occurs as the fingers are flexed around the block, with the MCP joints kept in extension, stretches the tight intrinsic musculature. This exercise is useful in early swan neck deformities and in metacarpophalangeal flexion contractures.

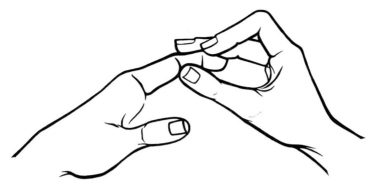

**FIGURE 34. Manually Assisted DIP Range of Motion.
(Stretching.)**
Flexion and extension of the DIP joint is assisted by the opposite hand.

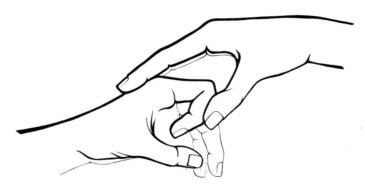

**FIGURE 35. Manually Assisted PIP Range of Motion.
(Stretching.)**
Flexion and extension of the PIP joint is assisted by the opposite hand.

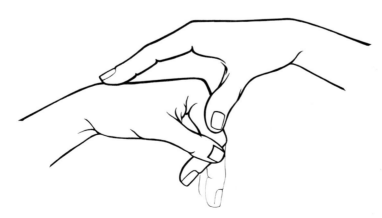

FIGURE 36. Manually Assisted MCP Range of Motion.
The MCP joint is flexed and extended with manual assistance of the opposite hand.

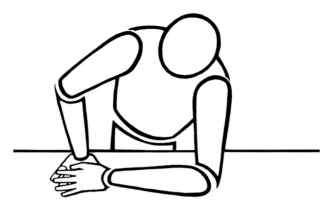

FIGURE 37.   Wrist Dorsiflexion.
(Assisted Stretching.)
The affected hand is placed on a table top and supported by the opposite hand. The body is gently leaned forward, creating leverage to stretch a contracture on the volar aspect of the wrist.

R — Rest
(See ADL.)

A — ADL
The scope of wrist and hand protection options includes the use of two hands whenever possible; carrying loads on large joints to protect smaller ones (a shoulder bag versus a hand grip on a purse); dividing packages and tasks into smaller burdens; building up and cushioning handles; using proper and efficient tools for tasks (sharp knives, power-driven pencil sharpeners); and pacing tasks to avoid overuse and joint or muscle tendon fatigue.[4,17,22,23]

P — Psychological Problems
Psychological problems related to the loss of hand function and the negative cosmetic impact of hand deformities or splints and braces may necessitate supportive therapy for optimal patient adjustment.

I — Immobilization
Thumb stabilizing splints provide good pain control while permitting useful thumb function in **osteoarthritis** and **de Quervain's** disease. These splints are recommended for daytime wear and can also be worn for comfort at night (Fig. 29).[11,17]

The *thumb IP joint* can become unstable in hyperextension with resultant loss of effective pinch. A plastic or metal splint can provide functional stability for this problem (Fig. 30).[11]

Tenosynovitis of the finger flexor tendons can often be relieved by a one-inch heavy elastic tubular sleeve worn over the PIP joints (thumb IP joint) during the day (Fig. 31).[11]

Function loss secondary to PIP hyperextension in **rheumatoid arthritis with swan-neck deformity** can be controlled with a splint similar to that used in the thumb IP joint.[11] When multiple adjacent PIP joints are involved, these splints can become quite cumbersome and may defeat their purpose—of improving function.

Wrist Splints. Prefabricated, commercially available, semi-rigid splints are available for night wear and can be effectively used in reducing night and often daytime manifestations of **carpal tunnel syndrome**. In many cases of carpal tunnel syndrome, night wear alone is all that is required. The splint should permit freedom of hand movement for function.

A more rigid wrist stabilizing splint for reduction of wrist movement and minimizing wrist strain (Fig. 38) is recommended for daytime wear in **rheumatoid arthritis** and related disorders, and can be worn for night comfort as well.[11,17]

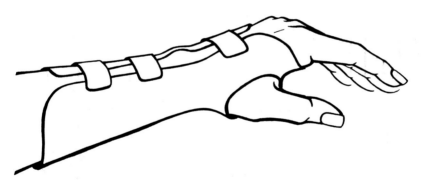

FIGURE 38. **Static Wrist Stabilizing (Working) Splint.**
This splint is a custom-molded thermo-labile plastic splint. It extends from distally just proximal to the distal palmar crease to the proximal one-third of the forearm. There is a wide aperture for thumb clearance. It is useful in arthritis of the wrist and to prevent hyperflexion and hyperextension of the wrist in the carpal tunnel syndrome.

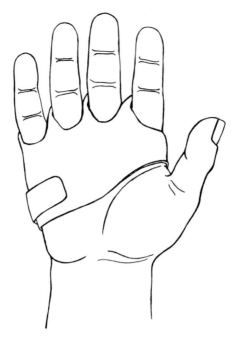

FIGURE 39.   Ulnar Deviation Splint.
This is a thermo-labile plastic custom-molded splint that extends from the distal one-third of the proximal phalanges to end just proximal to the distal creases. It is designed to permit only partial MCP flexion but full PIP and DIP motion. A vane on the ulnar side of each finger resists ulnar deviation. The thumb is free; the dorsal strap and Velcro closure hold the splint in place. This splint may improve function in patients with severe ulnar deviation. Its value in prophylaxis or correction of ulnar deviation is not established.

Ulnar deviation splints come in a variety of shapes (Fig. 39).[17] Their efficacy in preventing ulnar deviation is not established. Some patients appear to *benefit from improved hand function and lessened pain* when wearing such splints, and *this should be the only criteria* for recommending their use until such time as their efficacy for preventing deformity can be established.

It is extraordinarily rare for a patient to have such severe hand and/or wrist involvement as to require their total immobilization in a so-called *"pancake" splint.* Needless to say, the inability to grasp and pull up blankets at night is reason enough to condemn their casual prescription.

E — Education
The hand is an extremely complex structure and its relevance to almost all aspects of daily living demands detailed explanations, demonstrations (and return demonstrations by the patient), and follow-up to see that all aspects of care are understood and performed as prescribed.

S — Socioeconomic
The socioeconomic impact from loss of hand function can be disastrous. Early and adequate supportive therapy should be instituted.

5. UPPER BACK DISORDERS

Disorders of the spine, both anatomically and clinically, can be segregated into dorsal and lumbar (lumbosacral) disorders. Many problems of the upper dorsal and interscapular area are referred from the cervical spine and associated with focal muscle spasm or trigger areas, also on a referred basis. Treatment of such problems should address both the neck and the areas of referral as well as any disorders related to the dorsal spine per se.

In children and young adults, **scoliosis** is the most common source of problems, with **Scheuermann's epiphysitis** and **dorsal kyphosis** a close second.[105] Scoliosis, unless severe, is usually painless in youth and is treated symptomatically in adults (or surgically, if progressive or relentlessly painful). Postural instructions and corrective exercises are of limited value in correcting or preventing deformity, but stretching and gentle conditioning help relieve annoying discomfort related to scoliosis.[27-29] **Scheuermann's epiphysitis** must be differentiated from ankylosing spondylitis because of its self-limiting nature and more benign prognosis. The value of postural instruction and conditioning in Scheuermann's has not been established but, like ankylosing spondylitis, the effort to minimize dorsal kyphosis by posture instruction and exercises seems warranted, and bracing has been demonstrated to reverse the dorsal kyphosis.[3,30,31]

The most common serious problem affecting the dorsal spine is a fracture secondary to **osteoporosis** in the postmenopausal female and in the chronic steroid-treated patient. Management of the acute problem consists of pain control measures and relies on a *dorsolumbar corset*, local ice and occasional benefit from TNS use in lieu of, or with, analgesic medications. Long-term management is medical (diet, calcium supplementation, vitamin D plus estrogens and fluorides) and an attempt to increase bone calcium deposition through *exercise*. Resumption of ambulation is made as soon as tolerated, and slow progression of back and neck conditioning is instituted. Specific back extension conditioning is deferred until adequate fracture healing (3 to 6 months) has occurred. It is important to note that exercises designed to strengthen the back extensor musculature can be stressful to the low back area and may initiate or exacerbate problems in this area.[32,33]

For the clinician, the most common important problem affecting the dorsal spine is ankylosing spondylitis and associated **spondyloarthropathies**. The management is medical, with emphasis on posture control to minimize dorsal kyphosis and a general stretching regimen to relieve stiffness. Again, although one could reason from the successful experience with *bracing* in Scheuermann's epiphysitis that bracing in ankylosing spondylitis should be useful for posture control, this has, in fact, not been demonstrated.[3,30,31] **Disseminated idiopathic skeletal hyperostosis (DISH)** should not be a problem other than the need to recognize its presence and to realize that stiffness (loss of back motion as distinct from soreness and stiffness or attempting to move) in the face of ankylosis cannot be relieved by exercise. Occasionally the disks and/or facets that remain unankylosed may suffer from strain at a fulcrum where residual motion remains, and these may require local treatment (e.g., ice or ice massage, gentle mobilization, ultrasound, rotary stretches, posture and ADL instruction) and/or nonsteroidal antiinflammatory drugs.

45

Dorsal discogenic disease with disk space narrowing and prominent anterior lipping is very common radiographically, but symptoms are surprisingly rare. **Facet joint arthritis** is an expected accompaniment of disk disorders, and both disk and facet dysfunction can be associated with pain in the mid-dorsal and paraspinal areas and/or in a specific radicular or costal distribution. These disorders are also managed with local treatment and nonsteroidal antiinflammatory drugs. A *dorsolumbar corset* can be useful in reducing associated discomfort (Fig. 40).

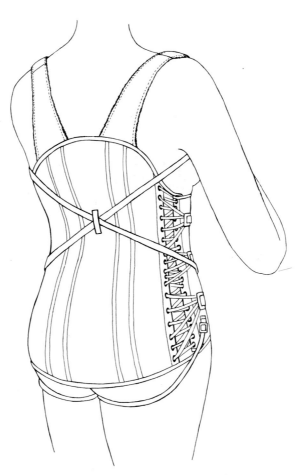

FIGURE 40.   **Thoraco-Lumbar Corset.**

This is a fabric corset with adjustable lacing and elastic components to permit snugness of fit. It is reinforced by stays to increase rigidity. This corset extends from beneath the lower curve of the buttocks to the mid-scapular area and is held in place superiorly by shoulder straps. The use of mesh fabric improves ventilation; however, in warm climates a long spinal (Taylor) brace may be preferred. These corsets are useful in generalized osteoporosis, in dorsal spinal compression fractures (regardless of etiology), and in painful osteoarthrosis of the dorsal or dorsolumbar spine.

The *dorsolumbar curve* area (T9 through L1) is, like the lower cervical spine and lumbosacral area, a region of postural strain. Problems here are similar to those in the dorsal spine except that pain and muscle spasm may be referred to the flanks and lateral pelvis and buttocks where local therapy should also be administered.[17]

T — Therapeutic Modalities

Ultrasound for facet joint pain, TNS for radicular pain, ice packs, and focal TNS (point finder) are often helpful pain control measures.

H — Hands-On

Mobilization in a graded fashion (segment-specific posterior-anterior) can relieve disk- and facet-related pain temporarily—from hours to days and occasionally definitively.[34] *Rib-referred* radicular pain can also be similarly benefited by local therapies and manual manipulation.[16,17] Acupressure—deep kneading manipulation of painful focal muscle spasm—can also help relieve pain.

E — Exercise

Stretching. Exercise to relieve discomfort includes rotary dorsolumbar stretches and extensor *automanipulations* (leaning back over a firmly rolled towel or arching over a towel or tennis ball placed on the floor just distal to the focal painful segment) (Figs. 41, 42).

Strengthening. Strengthening of the upper back commences from the prone position with pillows or a bolster supporting the abdomen and maintaining lumbar kyphosis to protect the low back. Single arm raises (antigravity exercise), single leg raises, then alternating arm-leg and bilateral arm, bilateral leg raises, are a useful progression (Figs. 43–46).[11,33,35] Weights of one to two pounds can be added to the wrists and ankles to increase the resistance. A *quadruped* (hands and knees) *posture* (Figs. 47, 48) can be used for similar exercises, and still more vigorous exercises (and therefore more stressful to the lumbar spine) can be performed with the *patient prone* with the abdomen directly on the mat without an intervening pillow.[11,33,35] This progression can be offered to patients with *ankylosing spondylitis*, *Scheuermann's epiphysitis* and *osteoporosis*. In the **osteoporosis patients**, particular *caution* must be observed before atempting to progress the patient, lest increased pain should result.

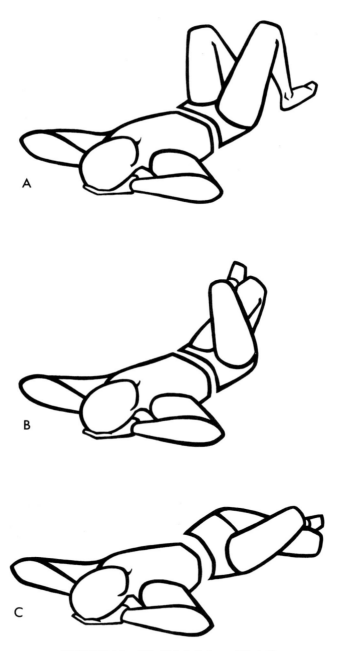

FIGURE 41. Hip-Pelvis Internal Rotation.
(Active-Assisted Stretch of External Rotary Components of the Hip and
Lumbosacral Fascia.)
The patient is supine with knees flexed and feet flat on the floor. The foot of one leg
is placed on the outside of the opposite knee. The foot then helps to push the knee of the
internally rotating hip toward the floor. The patient's upper back and shoulders remain in
the starting position to permit maximum rotation at the hip and lumbosacral area.

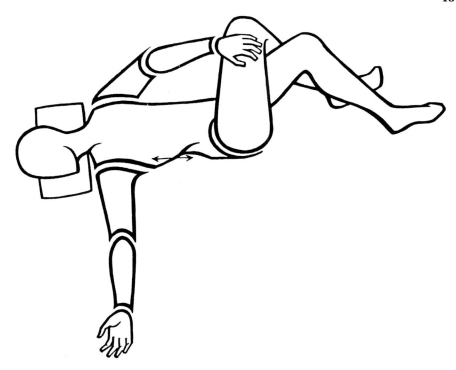

FIGURE 42.   Dorsolumbar Stretch.

The purpose of this exercise is to increase rotational mobility of the dorsolumbar spine and to increase suppleness during turning movements. The patient is instructed to lie flat on his back and do a gentle pelvic tilt to flatten the spine against the floor. The right leg is then crossed over the left with the right foot being placed over the outside of the left knee. The patient is instructed to do a ''log roll,'' moving the knees and shoulders together, until he is lying on the left side. The left hand is then placed over the right knee to keep it firmly in position and the patient slowly rolls the right shoulder back, turning the head to the right and extending the right hand as far as possible to the right. Once the maximum position is achieved he is to count to six and then, after completing the stretch, roll to the left side lying position, log roll back onto the back, uncross the legs, and repeat the exercise to the opposite side.

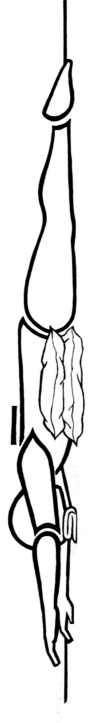

FIGURE 43. **Prone Single Arm Raise.**

The purpose of this exercise is to strengthen the back extensors, particularly upper dorsal and posterior scapular muscles. The patient is instructed to place two pillows under the abdomen and a small pillow or towel roll under the forehead. A pelvic tilt is performed and then both arms are stretched out on the floor in front of the patient's head. Maintaining the pelvic tilt, or the back flat, and keeping the forehead down, the patient raises the left arm a few inches off the floor and holds for a count of 10 to 20 or until the point of fatigue. The arm is slowly lowered and the opposite side is then exercised.

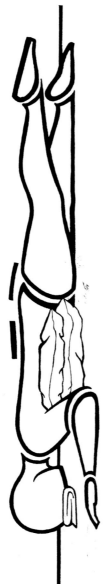

FIGURE 44. **Prone Single Leg Raise.**

The purpose of this exercise is to strengthen the gluteal and lumbar and hamstring muscles as well as to increase extension in the hips. The patient assumes a prone position with two pillows under the stomach and the forehead on a towel roll or small pillow. The hands are placed on either side of the head with the elbows bent. The left leg is slowly raised a few inches off the ground and held in that position for a count of 10 to 20 and then slowly lowered, and the exercise is repeated on the opposite side.

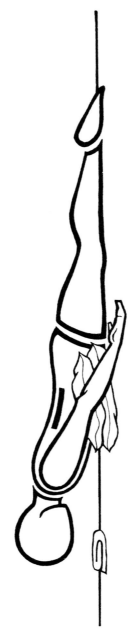

FIGURE 45. **Prone Upper Trunk Raise.**

The purpose of this exercise is to strengthen muscles in the upper back and scapular area. The patient assumes a prone position with two pillows under the abdomen and a small pillow or towel roll under the forehead. The arms are placed at the side, a pelvic tilt is performed, and with the chin tucked in the patient slowly raises his trunk and arms so that the chest rises about 3 inches above the floor. This is held for a count of 10 to 20 and repeated until mild fatigue is noted.

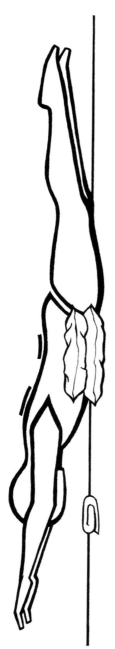

FIGURE 46. **Prone Bilateral Arm and Leg Raise.**
The purpose of this exercise is to strengthen the cervical, dorsal and lumbar extensors and scapular stabilizers. The patient is placed in a prone position with or without pillows under the abdomen and with or without a towel roll under the forehead, depending on comfort. Both arms and legs are simultaneously slowly raised a few inches off the ground and held for a count of 10 to 20. The exercise can be repeated until mild fatigue is experienced.

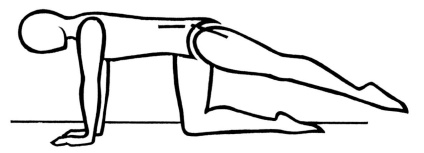

FIGURE 47.   Quadruped Single Leg Raise.

The purpose of this exercise is to strengthen the buttocks, posterior thigh and lower back muscles. The patient assumes the quadruped position, keeps the chin in and looks down at the floor. He then performs a pelvic tilt to flatten the back and then raises the left leg approximately 3 to 4 inches off the floor while avoiding extension in the low back. This position is held for a count of 10 to 20 and the leg is carefully returned to the start position. The exercise is then repeated on the opposite side, and the whole procedure can be repeated until mild fatigue is experienced.

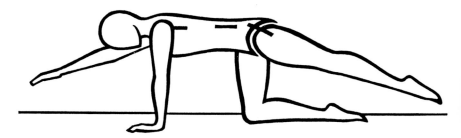

FIGURE 48.   Quadruped Contralateral Arm and Leg Raise.

The purpose is to simultaneously strengthen muscles on the opposite side of the spine to help improve coordination and control during reaching and athletic activities. The patient assumes the quadruped position, keeps the chin in, looking down at the floor, and then performs a pelvic tilt to flatten the lumbar spine. The left leg is raised about 3 to 4 inches off the floor and the right arm then is raised about 12 inches off the floor. This position is held for a count of 10 to 20 and then the patient relaxes to the start position and repeats the exercise on the opposite side. This exercise can be repeated until the point of gentle fatigue.

R — Rest

For pain control, this is essential in **acute spinal fracture**. Restful naps with emphasis on initiating the nap in an optimal posture (e.g., prone in ankylosing spondylitis, or side-lying for pain control) are beneficial in all chronic painful and inflammatory disorders.

A — ADL

The back protection and function enhancement of dorsal spine problems are no different, albeit generally less demanding, than those discussed in the next chapter on low back disorders.[11,36,37]

P — Psychological Problems

Psychological problems attendant with painful and chronic illness require appropriate consultation and management. The use of low-dose *"antidepressant"* drugs is often helpful in pain control and in particular when night pain disturbs sleep.[38,39]

I — Immobilization

Dorsolumbar corsets and braces are bulky and cumbersome and give modest support, but are usually acceptable for the pain they relieve. This is particularly apt to be true in patients with osteoporosis and recent overt or occult fractures.[31,40,41] Corsets are easier to fit than braces. Braces are cooler, but more expensive and more bulky than corsets. Braces come in two general types: the Taylor brace, which is essentially a rigid dorsolumbar corset with abdominal support, and the Jewett or CASH (chest-and-symphysis-hyperextension) brace, which applies pressure by means of sternal and pubic plates and counter-pressure dorsally to help maintain the upright posture.[40,41] By and large, a *dorsolumbar corset does the job* as well as a brace and is less formidable in terms of patient acceptance—especially if its intended use is short term (one to three months) (Fig. 40).

An elastic *"rib belt"* is useful for intercostal pain affecting the lower ribs and/ or an osteoporosis-associated rib fracture.

E — Education

Apply basic principles.

S — Socioeconomic

Apply basic principles.

6. LOW BACK DISORDERS

Low back pain as a rheumatological rehabilitative challenge is either a **spondyloarthropathy** or a discogenic disorder.[106] The former is managed as discussed under The Upper Back. Additional techniques to help relieve morning stiffness and to loosen up prior to more specific therapeutic exercises are hugging the knees and rocking back and forth while supine, or rocking back and forth on hands and knees (Figs. 49–51).[3,11,29,30]

The bulk of low back problems, and in fact the predominant cause of all socioeconomically important musculoskeletal problems, is *attributable to disk-facet related lumbar and lumbosacral disorders.*[42] Although radiographically (inclusive of CT and MRI) one can often identify pathology in these disk-related structures, clinically correlatable morphological change with pain is still lacking in the majority of painful lumbosacral conditions.[43–45] Specificity of radiography is greater but far from absolute in the presence of sciatic or femoral radiculopathies.[43–45] Therefore, it is difficult and necessarily arbitrary to make a precise clinical diagnosis, even though there are strong advocates for the specificity of various clinical diagnostic entities, ranging from psoas muscle spasm through sacroiliac subluxation to facet joint impingement and/or arthrosis and various disk bulges, herniations and fragment extrusions.[12,46] These various conditions suggest specific manipulative or traction strategies and have strong advocates, some consensus, and no convincing data to support assertions.[12,46] The author's bias will be revealed and the hope is given that newer technologies (MRI, more refined CT, and more sophisticated electrodiagnostic procedures) will provide answers.[107]

In the treatment of low back pain with or without radiculopathies, there is a consensus that *rest*, preferably in bed, is a safe and reliable initial strategy.[12,47–49]

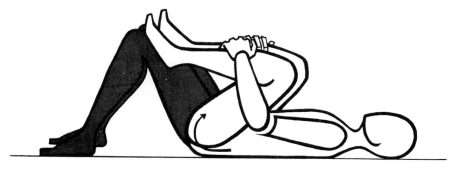

FIGURE 49.   Bilateral Knee-Chest.
(Active Stretch of the Lumbar and Gluteal Fascia.)
This exercise is usually introduced after the alternating knee-chest exercise shown in Figure 55. The bilateral knee-chest exercise is a somewhat more vigorous stretch of the lumbosacral fascia. Care must be taken that both legs are lowered carefully to the starting position with knees flexed. Initially, this should be done with one leg lowered at a time. If a knee is painful, the hands should be placed on the distal thigh behind the knee.

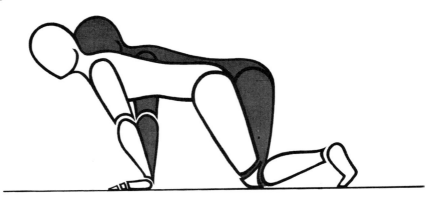

FIGURE 50.   Kneeling-Rocking.
(Shoulder Spine Hip Flexion-Extension Stretching.)
    The patient kneels on the floor or on a bed and rocks back on his haunches and forward over his hands and alternately places his back in an arched or sway position. This is an excellent "loosening-up" exercise for patients with generalized morning stiffness.

In the absence of radiculopathy, bedrest for one to two days often suffices.[50] Following and/or accompanying rest, there are currently two schools of approaches to therapeutic exercises. The traditional school follows the teaching of Williams, and recommends a basic series of *flexion exercises* and places strong emphasis on abdominal muscle strengthening.[31] This is extended by self-manipulation rocking in a supine flexion exercise, as recommended by Macnab (Fig. 49).[51] In contradistinction is the approach based on an attempt to reposition the posterior disk bulge anteriorly by *extension maneuvers*, exercise and postural strategies. This approach was first advocated by Cyriax and recently popularized by McKenzie (Figs. 52–53).[46,52]

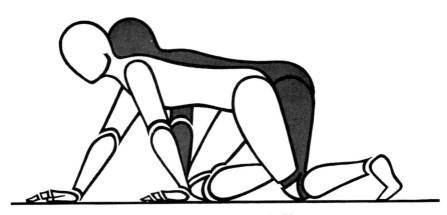

FIGURE 51.   Crawling in Place.
(Shoulder-Spine-Hip Flexion-Extension Stretching.)
    This is a second phase of the previous exercise (Fig. 50). The patient alternately reaches with an arm and a leg in a crawling-in-place motion or actually crawls. This provides a controlled stretch to the shoulders and hips and spine and serves as a mobilizing exercise to relieve morning stiffness and as a prelude to more vigorous exercise therapy.

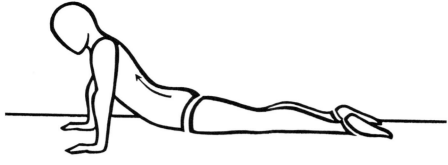

FIGURE 52.   Press-Ups.

The purpose of this exercise is to squeeze posteriorly displaced intraannular disk material into a more anterior position. It also provides a backward extension stretch to maintain spinal mobility. The patient is instructed to lie on his abdomen with the palms placed under the shoulders in a push-up position. He is told to relax the back, buttocks and legs, keeping the legs slightly apart. He then uses the arms to push the chest and head upward with the head held in a chin-in position. The exercise should be performed smoothly, under control, with the action coming from the arms while passive extension occurs in the lumbar spine to create a pincer movement of the posterior aspects of the vertebral bodies against the posteriorly protruding annular discal tissues. The up position is held for a slow count of three and then the patient returns to the start position on the count of two, and the exercise is repeated 10 to 12 times with hourly repetitions if the patient is on a bedrest program. The exercise is also performed before and after any flexion exercises are introduced to the treatment regimen.

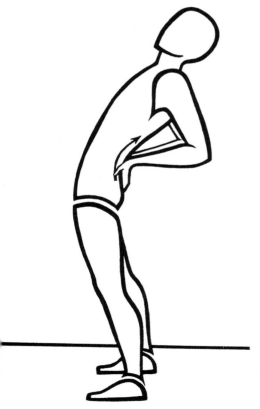

FIGURE 53.   Standing Extension. (Back Bends.)

The purpose of this exercise is to squeeze bulging discal material anteriorly away from the spinal cord and nerves. The patient is instructed to assume a comfortable stance with the feet about shoulder width apart. The hands are placed at waist level on either side of the back to serve as a fulcrum at the lumbosacral area over which the back is to bend. The knees are kept straight, the chin is maintained in a chin-in position. The spine is relaxed and the patient bends backward in a slow, deliberate manner while saying "pres-sure on, pressure off" or "one-two-three, one-two-three." The exercise is repeated 10 to 12 times and is performed after transfers such as from sitting to standing, getting in and out of a car, after working at a desk or before and after doing chores and other household or vocational activities.

Obviously, there is more than one way to skin a cat, and for some, one way may be better than another. We have employed techniques of both schools successfully, using the criteria of McKenzie as guidelines.[52] In the final analysis, rest and time, good posture and body mechanics, and gradual reconditioning are the keys to successful back rehabilitation, even for the majority of patients suffering from complicating sciatic or femoral radiculopathies confirmed by EMG, myelogram, CT or MRI.[47,48,53,54,108]

T — Therapeutic Modalities

Use of various modalities described below in *spondyloarthropathies* is generally not rewarding. In discogenic disorders, the use of *focal injections of steroids* (2–5 mg of triamcinolone hexacetonide in 3–5 ml of 1% lidocaine) can help relieve pain when injected into *tender entheses* (the posterior superior iliac spine and/or posterior iliac crest areas) and the anatomical area of locally *tender facet joints* (direct fluoroscopic visualization is occasionally necessary from the standpoint of clinical evaluation of the diagnostic strategy, as well as to determine precisely the site injected). The local injection of 3–5 ml of 1% lidocaine into areas of palpable **muscle induration** and tenderness (''**muscle spasm**'') can relieve pain for prolonged periods and occasionally is a definitive therapy.[19]

Local *ice massage, cold packs, spray and stretch* and *focal TNS* (*point finder*) and, almost interchangeably, *ultrasound* are useful pain control modalities. TNS can be readily administered on a home program. In more chronic cases, a moist compress or a heating pad provides comfort and may obviate the need for medication. In this connection, one can also consider the use of over-the-counter *counterirritant ointments* (e.g., back rubs).[9,10,55–59]

TNS is an extremely useful pain control measure for **radiculopathies** and generally a less helpful measure for back pain per se.[7,8]

Pelvic traction is unpredictable as a pain control measure but should be considered in older patients with back pain, with or without radiculopathy unresponsive to bedrest and other modalities.[47] Traction is typically administered by a machine-driven traction apparatus creating a tractive force of one third to one half of the patient's weight with the patient on a friction-free table. The treatment sessions last for 20 to 30 minutes and if successful the method rarely requires more than 10 sessions one to three days apart for symptomatic control.[47,60] Pelvic traction can occasionally exacerbate symptoms of back pain or radiculopathy.[46]

Inverted or vertical traction devices are rapidly losing their popularity. This is probably attributable to a lack of convincing evidence of efficacy, although the rationale for their use seems plausible.[61,62] Inverted traction causes some risk of elevation of blood pressure, food regurgitation, and retinal detachment.[12]

H — Hands-On

Spray-and-stretch for focal muscle spasm and deep kneading massage ''*acupressure*'' over these areas are generally acceptable pain control techniques. *Manipulation* is another story.[12,101] In short, there are a variety of gentle vibratory ''mobilization'' techniques that can be administered. These are typically done manually with AP mobilization of the vertebral bodies by pressure on the spine and transverse processes and in a rotary lumbosacral pattern, in an attempt to provide pain relief and to facilitate exercise and functional activity progression.[12,34] Alternatively, use of brief muscle contraction and relaxation and the related ''muscle energy'' technique provide easily administered methods that *in some instances can be self-administered* by the patient for stretching and pain control.[20,21,63]

Proof of efficacy for these methods is lacking. However, the likelihood of harm is slim when these gentle maneuvers are performed with reasonable care, and they seem to provide a satisfying aspect of ''hands-on'' care to both patient and therapist.[34]

The real rub comes from *manipulation*. Whether or not a disk protrusion can be replaced, a facet joint displacement realigned, or a nerve root compression relieved by a *high-speed thrust maneuver* remains a question.[12] Studies to date at best support a reduction of duration of symptomatology but no long-term outcome benefit.[12] It seems clear that the high-speed thrusting manipulation, which carries a risk of fracture or disk extrusion, is capable of harm and at best gives short-term pain control but does not affect the ultimate outcome of disk-related disorders.[12] Nonetheless, for those patients who obtain prompt relief from these maneuvers (or learn to do them themselves when their back is ''out''), manipulation therapy remains a popular and attractive, but all too often nonmedical, alternative therapy.

E — Exercise

The *Williams flexion exercises* are tried and true, or at least time-honored.[32] Successful exercise must respect pain and a time course for healing of injured tissue. A gentle *pelvic tilt* maneuver with knees bent and the spine flat in the supine position is usually the first well-tolerated exercise for a patient with an acute episode of back pain (Fig. 54). This is not initially performed as a raised, low back, bridging

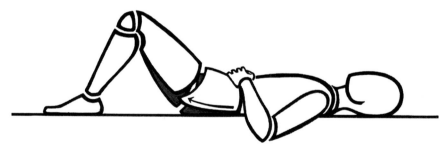

FIGURE 54. Pelvic Tilt.
(Active Stretch of the Lumbar Fascia, with Terminal Isometric Hold for Gluteal Strengthening.)

The patient is supine with the lumbar spine flattened against the floor or mat and both knees flexed and feet planted. The hands are placed over the lower abdomen in order to help reinforce the flattened lumbar spine position. The pelvis is tilted posteriorly by contraction of the abdominal muscles (this is perceived as a sensation of the anterior superior iliac spines moving away from the hands placed on the abdomen as well as by a sense of lifting in the sacro-coccygeal region). The gluteal muscles are tightened during this movement, and a firm isometric contraction at the termination of the full pelvic rotation or pelvic tilt adds an isometric strengthening of the gluteal muscles to the stretch of the lumbosacral fascia. This exercise is useful as an initial exercise in a back reconditioning program because it is usually well tolerated. It also provides a means of creating an awareness of the flattening of the lumbar spine that occurs during posterior tilting of the upper pelvis. It is an effective exercise to relieve discomfort associated with chronic stiffness in the low back or stiffness that is aggravated by poor sleeping or sitting posture.

maneuver, as this is frequently painful in the early convalescent stage. Gentle alternating *knee-to-chest* stretches (Fig. 55) and a supine *isometric abdominal strengthening* exercise (Fig. 56) held up to 40 seconds can be added as pain control is achieved.[11,32,33,35]

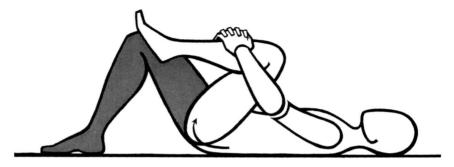

FIGURE 55. Knee Flexion-Alternating Knee-Chest.
(Manually Assisted Stretch of Knee Extensors and Lumbosacral Fascia.)
The patient is supine with both knees flexed. Alternately, one knee and then the other is brought to the chest, with flexion manually assisted by grasping the anterior surface of the tibia. This exercise is also a gentle stretch of the lumbosacral fascia and can be used early in the recovery from discogenic disease and lumbosacral strain. The hands should be placed behind the knee to avoid aggravating any knee joint disorder.

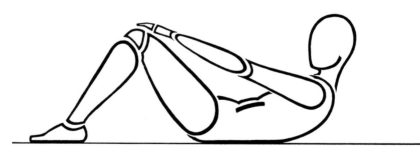

FIGURE 56. Abdominal Isometric Exercise.
(Strengthening of Abdominal Musculature.)
This is exclusively a strengthening exercise but is placed here because it is a key exercise in a back reconditioning program and is usually introduced after pelvic tilt and knee-chest exercises. The patient is supine with the knees flexed and the feet flat. Keeping the lumbar spine flat, he/she attempts to lift the upper dorsal spine and head so that the hands reach to or over the knees. This position is held initially for a count of six to provide an adequate isometric strengthening stimulus. Ultimately this is increased to a count of 40 or to a point of fatigue just short of that which would preclude a controlled resumption of the supine position. The patient exhales or counts out loud during the isometric contraction (as in all isometric exercises).

The hierarchy of exercise that follows is arbitrary, but *a step-wise progression of exercise* seems to facilitate the reconditioning process and includes supine, knee-bent, gentle, pelvic side-to-side rotations (Fig. 57); hamstring stretches (Fig. 58); heel cord stretches (Fig. 59); lumbosacral stretches (Fig. 41); quadriceps and gluteal conditioning (Figs. 60, 61); and finally progressive back extensor strengthening as outlined in Chapter 5, Upper Back.[11,33,35]

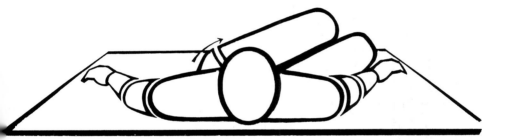

FIGURE 57.   **Beginning Pelvic Rotation.**
The purpose of this exercise is to stretch the lumbosacral and buttocks muscles in a diagonal pattern. The patient lies supine with the knees bent and the feet on the floor. The hands are placed at the side and, with the knees kept together, the hips are slowly rotated to the right as far as required to get a gentle stretch. This position is held for a slow count of six. The patient relaxes, returns to the starting position, and repeats the exercise on the opposite side. The exercise can be repeated three to five times until an optimum stretch is achieved.

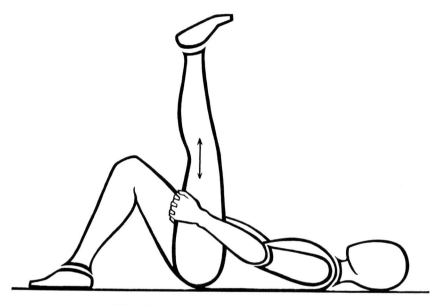

FIGURE 58.   Supine Hamstring Stretch.

The purpose of this exercise is to stretch the hamstring muscles. The patient is instructed to lie down supine with both knees bent and perform a mild pelvic tilt to maintain a flat lumbar spine. The hands are placed behind the left knee and the neck and shoulders are relaxed. The thigh is then grasped with both hands and the leg slowly straightened until a tolerable stretch is experienced in the back of the knee. The stretch can be accentuated by dorsiflexing the foot. The stretch is held for a slow count of six and then the leg is allowed to relax. The exercise is then repeated on the opposite side. The exercise can be repeated three to five times until an optimal stretch is attained. Additional stretching can often be achieved if the patient holds the leg in the fully stretched position and pushes firmly against the resistance of his hands for a count of three and then relaxes the leg and "takes up slack." This contract-relax mechanism can be facilitory to the stretching process.

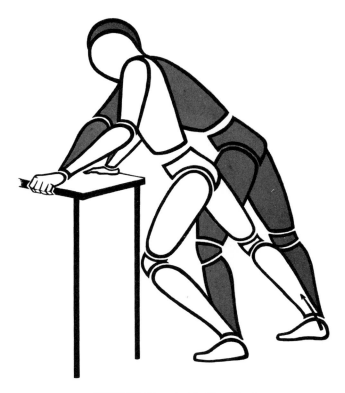

FIGURE 59. Ankle Dorsiflexion.
(Active-Assisted Gastrocnemius-Soleus-Achilles Tendon Stretch.)
This is a vigorous stretch of the ankle plantar flexors. The patient stands before a table and extends the affected leg posteriorly. He then flexes the opposite knee while attempting to keep the foot of the affected ankle flat on the ground. By leaning toward the table, the ankle plantar flexors are stretched.

**FIGURE 60. Partial Deep Knee Bend.
(Dynamic Endurance Exercise for the
Quadriceps and Gluteal Muscle.)**

This is a dynamic endurance conditioning exercise that is placed here because it is the appropriate next step in a sequence of increasingly more vigorous back reconditioning exercises. The exercise as shown shows the patient utilizing the back of a chair for support. While partially lowering and raising himself, the spine is kept flattened and the movements are controlled. This exercise is best initiated with the patient standing with his back to a wall and his heels three or four inches away from the wall. He then slides up and down utilizing the wall as a support. In this technique he learns to flatten his entire spine against the wall and thereby to reinforce a posture which puts minimal stress on the lumbosacral fascia and underlying structures. The exercise also serves to remind the patient to assume the proper standing posture and use flexion of the knees and hips or a squatting posture to retrieve low-lying articles or fallen objects. The exercise is repeated initially three to five times and progresses until approximately 40 knee bends can be accomplished rhythmically and under control.

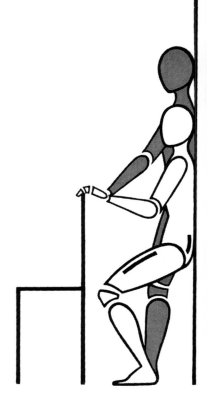

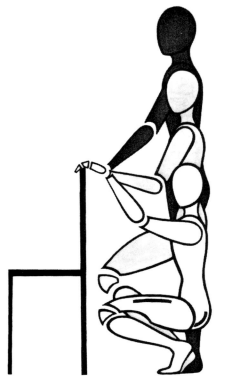

**FIGURE 61. Deep Knee Bends.
(Dynamic Endurance For Quadriceps and
Gluteal Muscles.)**

This is a more vigorous exercise than the preceding one and further helps to prepare patients to retrieve objects from the floor as well as to increase their overall physical fitness. Hip and knee and occasionally ankle problems may preclude the use of the deep knee bend.

When these exercises are safely and comfortably performed, specific conditioning for sports can be commenced and a therapeutic *regimen simplified into a 5- to 10-minute maintenance routine* that can also be used as part of *warm-up and cool-down for sports* activities.

Low back pain patients usually tolerate *swimming* (if they are competent swimmers), *walking*, and *bicycling* (upright touring position with short hip-to-crank radius, i.e., incomplete hip-knee extension with the pedal down, to minimize pelvic rotation).[64] Most patients can return to *golf and tennis* if mindful of minimizing excessive spinal rotation or extension, and many can resume *jogging*, provided they use good footwear and jog on a firm but cushioned surface. *Skiing*, both Nordic and downhill, is surprisingly well-tolerated, with reasonable care to ski in control under optimal conditions and to avoid rope tows.

R — Rest

Literally, the back bone of acute back care is rest. *Side-lying with a pillow between drawn-up knees and supine positioning with bent knees* supported on a bolster or a gatched hospital bed (with a *firm but not rigid mattress*) are the most comfortable postures and are associated with the least intradiscal pressures.[42,49,65] Bedrest can be unsuccessful if *techniques for transferring in and out of bed* are not carefully taught (Figs. 62–64).[11,37] *Traction in bed* has no demonstrable value.[11,60] Rest in bed should be continued until only mild analgesic medication is required (typically one to three days in the absence of radiculopathy) and any radiculopathy has stabilized, or better, is clearly regressing.[50] In addition to the sensory and motor examination, the end points of straight leg Lasègue's and Ely's tests in terms of the angle at which radicular symptoms are precipitated are very useful guidelines for assessing the status of radicular irritation and the timing of resumption of gradually increased activity levels.[38,54,66]

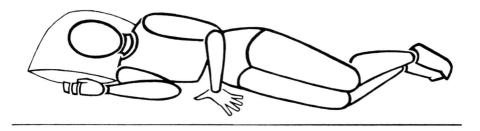

FIGURE 62.   Side Lying or "Hook" Lying Position.
(Initial Step in Transferring from Lying to Standing Position.)
The patient is generally most comfortable in this position with the hips and knees moderately flexed, the lumbar spine flat, and the neck supported. A firm mattress is essential for support during transfer. The patient should be close to the edge of the mattress.

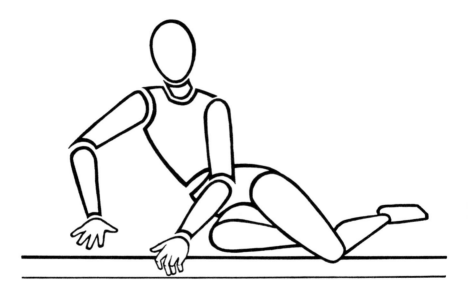

FIGURE 63. **Semi-Seated Supported Position.**
(Step 2 in Transferring from Lying to Standing.)
Using both arms for support, the body is carefully moved into a semi-seated position.

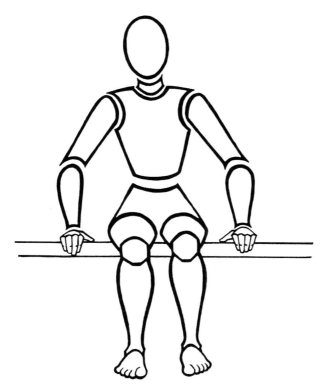

FIGURE 64. **Seated Manually Supported Position.**
(Step 3 in Transfer Process.)

With careful arm support the patient has lowered first one leg and then the other so that he assumes a sitting position. From this position the patient keeps his back firm and slides to the edge of the bed. He then carefully partially rotates to one side, sliding his feet to the floor one at a time, the outermost foot first. If able, the patient should be taught to move from the semi-sitting to the sitting posture in one smooth motion by simultaneously easing both legs (held together) over the edge of the mattress. With one hand supported on the mattress and the lumbosacral angle kept flat or slightly swayed back, he rises in a controlled manner to assume the standing posture, placing his weight on the "good" leg first. The entire process is reversed in a stepwise fashion on returning to bed.

A — ADL

Squatting or kneeling lifting techniques; careful *reaching techniques*; proper *sitting with firm lumbar support* (Fig. 13) on a knee-height firm seat; proper adjustment of seating in work areas and automobile driving; adjustment of heel height for leg length discrepancies; techniques for dressing and undressing and arising from a bed, chair or floor; use of reachers and long-handled shoe horns and slip-on shoes (Figs. 65, 66); use of dollies and wheeled luggage carriers and carts (for transporting packages, briefcases, etc.); techniques for bed-making, sweeping and mopping; pacing of activities to avoid strains from work or leisure activities—all require thoughtful appraisal, instruction in technique, and appropriate modification as recovery ensues.[11,36,37,42,48,64,65,67]

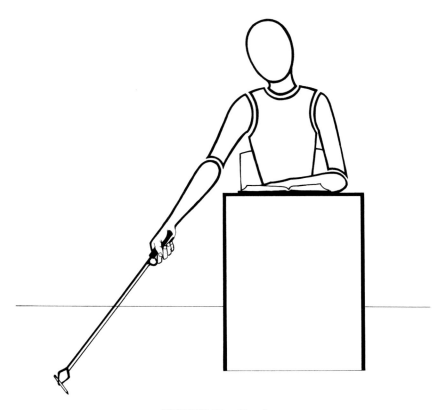

FIGURE 65.   **Reacher.**

This is one of several similar devices that permit patients sufficient grasp or reach to compensate for inability to bend down to recover dropped objects or to obtain objects from what would otherwise be inaccessible storage space.

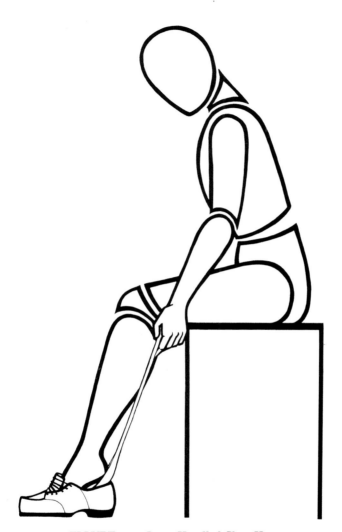

***FIGURE 66.*   Long-Handled Shoe Horn.**

A simple but too often overlooked device that can substitute independence and comfort in dressing for agony and the need for assistance. This long-handled shoe horn may be useful for patients with neck, back, hip or knee-joint distress. Note that elastic shoelaces, which do not require tying, will stretch sufficiently to permit insertion of the foot but provide enough tension to hold the shoe in place.

P — Psychological Problems

Back pain constitutes the largest diagnostic category for admission to pain control centers.[100] This includes failed surgery (often multiple operations),[109] drug abuse, and otherwise failed medical and nonallopathically managed patients. Good management and *early psychosocial intervention* should prevent the majority of chronic pain patients from requiring a trial of comprehensive pain center therapies. The *pain center treatments* include conventional diagnostic and therapeutic maneuvers, typically exhausting the possibilities of TNS, epidural or intrathecal steroid therapies and facet joint injections and/or deafferentation procedures, all of which can be accomplished prior to pain center admission.[48,53,55]

Current pain center programs typically utilize group therapies and individual psychotherapy with biofeedback, guided imagery, and other forms of hypnotherapy for pain control.[25,48,53,68] More importantly, they can create a psychotherapeutic environment and an opportunity for restructuring attitudes and adaptations to chronic pain. They can permit the patient and the pain to coexist in a lifestyle that is productive and positive for the patient. Outcomes from various configurations of pain center management profiles (e.g., hospital in-patient; partial in-patient—motel plus OPD—and ambulatory care) and durations of treatment of 3 to 8 weeks are such that the optimal configuration and mix of therapies and of patients is not yet determined, and many so-called pain centers are poorly staffed and poorly supervised.

Drug addiction and/or drug abuse and litigation and compensation issues clearly negatively bias outcome from any therapeutic endeavors and constitute the basis for the majority of failures in pain management.[48,53,54,68]

I — Immobilization

Bracing and corsetting for **spondyloarthropathies** have not been demonstrated to be helpful for pain or postural control.

In **acute discogenic syndromes**, most patients will obtain significant pain control with a *simple elastic abdominal binder*, especially if it is *reinforced with a heat-molded plastic lumbar support* that can be inserted into a sleeve in the back of the corset.[58] Typically, corsets are worn day and night for a few days and then daily for a few weeks, and are then gradually discontinued. A regimen for discontinuing a corset consists of wearing it in the afternoons when fatigue develops, while driving, and during unusual activities, and, finally, wearing it only during heavy activities until ultimately it is discontinued over a period of a month or so.

More substantial support can be provided with a *lumbosacral corset, preferably utilizing three straps* and semi-rigid posterior and lateral stays (Fig. 67).[11,40,41,69] A *brace* has the advantage of being cooler than a corset and is more durable, but

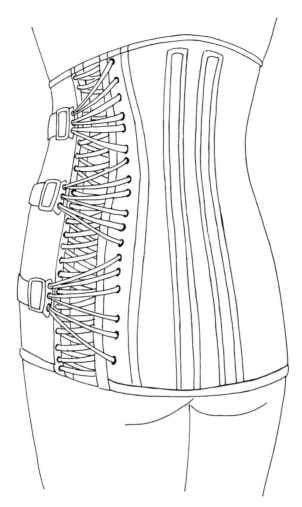

***FIGURE 67.* Lumbosacral Corset or Belt.**
This is a fabric corset that has adjustable lacing for snugness and is reinforced laterally and posteriorly by flexible or rigid stays or both. The "belt" is essentially a "male corset," more rigidly stayed posteriorly and usually designed with lateral lacing. Rigid stays are most efficient in restricting lateral motion but reduce comfort and ease of fitting. This corset should extend just above the lower ribs and anchor beneath the curve of the buttocks. Firm approximation of all surfaces and abdominal compression are essential to the proper fit. Rib compression may be painful and necessitate corset modification. There should be sufficient space so that compression of the upper anterior thigh does not occur when sitting. The lumbosacral corset or belt is indicated for moderate to severe low back pain, with or without radiculopathy.

they tend to be bulky and more expensive. For the laborer or athlete, a sturdy brace can provide a measure of support during vigorous activity (Fig. 68).[69]

A 2-inch to 4-inch belt of heavy elastic webbing (a *sacroiliac belt*) worn between the iliac crests and the hips can sometimes produce sufficient restriction of lumbosacral or sacroiliac motion in addition to providing lower abdominal support to minimize low back pain and strain. Lateral femoral nerve palsy is a not uncommon complication of sacroiliac belts.

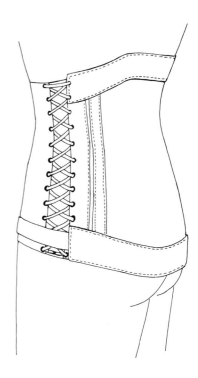

FIGURE 68. **Lumbosacral Chair-Back Brace.**

This is a metal and leather or plastic brace. A pelvic band is located between the iliac crest and the greater trochanter and is attached by posterior and lateral upright steel struts to a low thoracic band. Firm abdominal compression is applied through the laced front "corset" attachment. This brace is heavier and more rigid but cooler than a corset. Close fitting of the pelvic and thoracic bands is crucial for stability and comfort. It is indicated in refractory painful low back problems. Its chief advantage, other than durability, may be in restricting lateral flexion.

E — Education

The whole gamut of therapies and back protective strategies must be fully understood by the patient so that adherence to the regimen prescribed can be anticipated. The word "disk" conveys an impression of the inevitability of surgery, and the word "degenerative" speaks for itself. Patients must be made more aware of their own recuperative potential and of their all-important role in making the recuperation possible.[110]

S — Socioeconomic

As in all painful musculoskeletal problems, and particularly with reference to low back pain—the premier socioeconomic and health care burden of working adults—all relevant factors must be considered early and constructive corrective measures implemented expeditiously.[38,53,54,66,68,111]

7. HIP DISORDERS

When your patient says, "My hip hurts," and points to the buttock or lateral upper thigh, it may well be that the hip is at fault. More often it will be the lumbar spine and/or a trochanteric bursa. If the patient points instead to the groin, it may be a lumbosacral pain referral, but if there is pain at the extremes of hip motion and, even more revealing, restriction of hip motion plus tenderness anteriorly over the joint capsule, then the hip joint is almost surely at fault. Finally, the patient may complain of knee pain when the hip is actually at fault.

Regardless of etiology, **hip joint disease** is treated pharmacologically with nonsteroidal antiinflammatory drugs and occasional intraarticular steroid injections. Regardless of etiology, if either the *submedius or submaximus trochanteric bursa* is irritated, local steroid injection into the bursa may dramatically reduce discomfort, often for months at a time.[70,71]

From a rehabilitative standpoint, therapy directed to hip joint disease will consist of relief of joint strain—by correction of *leg length discrepancy* with a heel lift and/or use of a cane or crutches (Fig. 69A, B). It will include exercise to maintain hip musculature strength and mobility. If the trochanteric bursal irritation is asso-

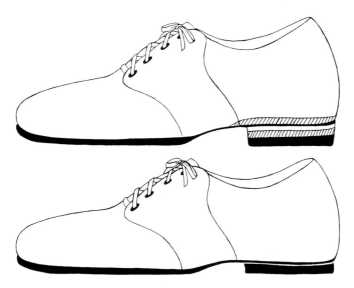

FIGURE 69A,B. **Shoe-Heel Lift (Leg Length) Correction.**
69A.   A ⅛ to ¼ inch correction can be applied inside or outside the heel. A combination of ¼ inch inside and ¼ inch outside the heel allows for a ½ inch correction. This usually does not cause forefoot stress and obviates the necessity to provide additional sole thickness and weight.
68B.   Removal of ¼ inch from the opposite heel is shown. This combination of ½ inch added to one shoe and ¼ inch removed from the other shoe permits a total correction of ¾ inch with good cosmesis, little added shoe weight, and no stressful foot positioning.

ciated with a *tight fascia lata* (positive Ober's sign), specific stretches directed to the problem can help relieve discomfort and minimize recurrences—if the exercises can be performed without increasing pain, muscle spasm and further restriction of mobility (Figs. 70, 71).[49]

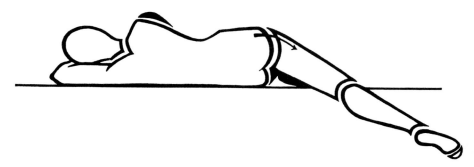

FIGURE 70.   Advanced Side-Lying Fascia Lata Stretch.

The purpose of this exercise is to stretch the gluteus medius and tensor fascia lata muscles. The patient lies on his side on the edge of the bed and bends the bottom knee toward the chest. The top leg is held in a straightened position and then allowed to dangle over the edge of the bed to create a gravity-assisted stretch to the lateral thigh musculature. The leg is held in the stretch position for a count of six and then returned to the start position. The exercise can be performed on the opposite side when indicated and can be repeated two to three times until optimal stretch is attained. The patient is cautioned to avoid arching the back during the exercise and to discontinue the exercise if pain on the outer upper thigh is increased.

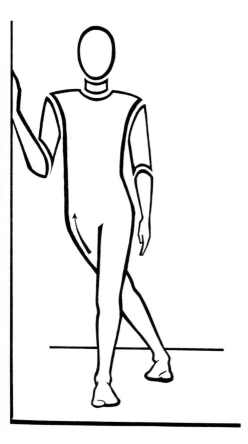

FIGURE 71. Standing Fascia Lata Stretch.

The purpose of this exercise is to stretch the fascia lata and gluteal muscles on the lateral side of the upper thigh. The patient is instructed to stand with his feet apart and the side to be stretched (right side) is positioned 1 foot away from the wall. The left leg is then crossed in front of the right and placed about 1 foot in front of the right foot with the toes parallel to the wall. With the right hand on the wall and the shoulders kept parallel to the floor, the patient leans toward the wall until a stretch is experienced in the right upper lateral thigh. The stretch should be held for a slow count of six and then the patient pushes back to the start position. This exercise can be repeated three to five times until an optimal stretch is experienced.

The last resort of hip joint disease salvage is surgical. The decision for surgery is a failure of medical management to impact favorably on pain and quality of life for the individual hip-disease sufferer, not the extent of x-ray changes per se, except in the case of early ischemic necrosis, when surgical intervention should be considered before collapse of the femoral head is obvious.[72-74]

T — Therapeutic Modalities

The usual trial of warm and cold compresses as well as soaking in a tub for pain control should be provided and are usually helpful prior to exercise. A whirlpool agitator can be a soothing adjunct. TNS occasionally gives sufficient benefit and pain control to justify the nuisance of being attached to wires and electrodes.

H — Hands-On

Manual distraction of the hip and stretching it through the available range of motion can relieve discomfort temporarily and may facilitate subsequent exercises to help restore mobility and strength.[16]

E — Exercise

Stretching. Stretching consists first of gentle stretches to maintain and then restore maximal mobility. Stretches are introduced first into flexion, then abduction, external and internal rotation, extension and adduction, in order to minimize pain and overcome significant tightness (Figs. 57, 72–75).[11,22]

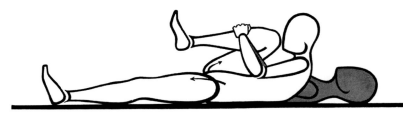

FIGURE 72. **Hip Flexion.**
(Active, Manually Assisted Stretch of the Extensors During Flexion with Simultaneous Stretch of the Hip Flexors on the Opposite Extended Side.)
The patient is supine. While keeping one leg fully extended on the floor or a mat, the opposite leg is flexed and assisted to the maximum flexion with the hands placed over the tibia. In some patients this may create stress at the knee joint, and the hands are then placed behind the distal femur. Neck and upper spine flexion augment the stretch throughout the entire spine. This exercise is a more vigorous knee flexion, hip flexion, and lumbosacral flexion stretch than that shown in Figure 55.

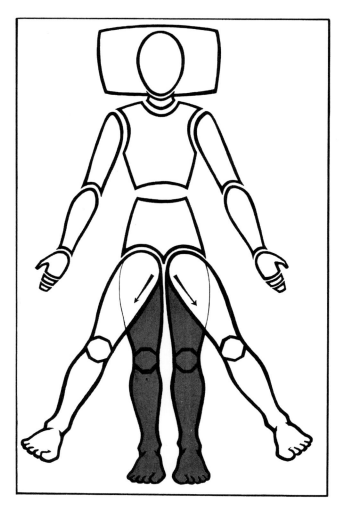

FIGURE 73. Hip Abduction-Adduction.
(Active Stretch of Adductors.)

The patient is supine with gravity eliminated. The legs are moved away from the midline and then returned in a series of stretching motions. This can be done alternately on one side and then the other or bilaterally. The use of a smooth gliding surface such as a powder board or performance of this exercise in water can facilitate the stretching. If performed unilaterally, crossing one leg over the other, the exercise can serve as a hip abductor stretch.

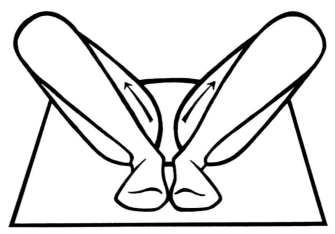

FIGURE 74.   Hip External Rotation Stretch.

The purpose of this exercise is to stretch the adductors and internal rotators of the hips. The patient is instructed to lie on his back with a gentle pelvic tilt to keep the back flattened against the floor. Both knees are bent and the feet are placed side by side. The patient keeps the feet juxtaposed and gently spreads the knees apart until a stretch is experienced in the inner sides of the thighs. Once a tolerable stretch is achieved, the legs are held abducted and externally rotated for a count of three and then the exercise is repeated three to five times until an optimal stretch is achieved. The stretch can be intensified somewhat by slowly pushing against the inner sides of the thighs with the hands.

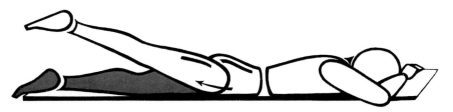

FIGURE 75.   Hip Extension.
(Active Extension Stretch of Hip and Lumbar Flexor Musculature.)

The patient is prone and alternately raises each leg as high as possible, returning it to the starting position before repeating the procedure on the opposite side. This exercise may be better tolerated if it is initially performed in the side-lying position. An isometric strengthening contraction at the extreme of hip extension can be added, if tolerated, at the end of the series of stretches. Back pain may preclude the use of this exercise.

Strengthening. Isometric hip abduction and extension exercises are usually well tolerated early, and strengthening in adduction and flexion can then be added (Figs. 76–78).

Recreational walking is not recommended, and jogging is best avoided. If pain permits, *cycling* with the seat and crank ratio reduced to minimize full hip and knee extension can often be successfully undertaken. *Swimming* is always the best all-around exercise for patients with joint disease. Many patients with hip osteoarthritis can not only swim but can play doubles tennis without aggravating their joint symptoms.

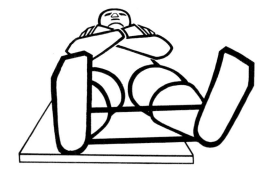

FIGURE 76. **Hip Abductor Strengthening. (Belt-Resisted Isometric.)**

The belt is looped over both ankles. The left hip abductors attempt a maximum contraction against the resistance of the belt. Strengthening stimuli occur in both the stabilizing extremity and the extremity being "exercised."

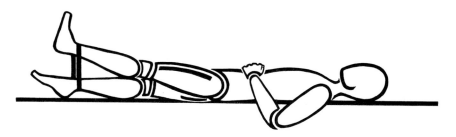

FIGURE 77. **Isometric Hip Extensor Strengthening.**

The patient lies in the supine position. The right heel and ankle are placed on top of three pillows or a partially inflated beach ball. The right knee is kept straight and the heel is pushed slowly and forcibly into the pillows, and this position is held as firmly as possible for a slow count of six. The exercise is then repeated on the opposite side if indicated, and the whole procedure repeated twice.

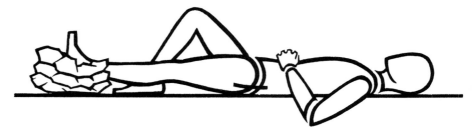

FIGURE 78. **Quadriceps and Opposite Gluteal-Hamstring Strengthening. (Belt-Resisted Isometric.)**
An elastic band or belt is looped over both ankles. In this exercise the quadriceps of the left or near leg is strengthened. There are simultaneous isometric contractions of the proximal hip extensors and hamstring musculatures in the stabilizing opposite leg. The isometric contraction is held for 6 seconds and the exercise is performed once to twice daily. Back pain may preclude use of this exercise.

R — Rest

Prone positioning at bedtime can help stretch tight hip flexor muscles, but one cannot stay in that position all night and should not try to do so. This posture can also aggravate associated lumbosacral discogenic problems. Sleeping in the *side-lying* position on the unaffected side with a pillow between the legs can relieve strain on a tight fascia lata and associated trochanteric bursae.

A — ADL

Pacing, arranging objects in daily use for easy accessibility, carrying small parcels, using *reachers* to retrieve fallen objects, and using a *cane* and/or *crutches*, can all help minimize hip strain. Correction of leg length discrepancies by *heel lifts* may also relieve discomfort (Fig. 69).

P — Psychological Problems

Psychological problems associated with pain, disability, and sexual dysfunction are commonly associated with hip joint disorders and need appropriate counseling.

I — Immobilization

Immobilization is rarely necessary, but in cases with extreme pain, as with sepsis, *longitudinal traction in bed* may help relieve discomfort until more specific therapy becomes effective.

E — Education

Apply basic principles.

S — Socioeconomic

Apply basic principles.

8. KNEE DISORDERS

The knee is a target joint for virtually all rheumatological disorders. Inflammatory effusions with characteristic circumferential joint margin tenderness comprise one group, and degenerative joint disease, traumatic arthropathies, and periarticular bursal and tendon inflammatory disorders with asymmetric and focal articular and/or periarticular tenderness make up another. Careful palpation and articular diagnostic maneuvering after a careful history usually can categorize the problem. Supportive or confirmatory diagnostic information are drawn from synovial analysis, other laboratory tests, x-rays, CT, MRI, and occasionally arthrography and arthroscopy.

The **inflammatory arthropathies** typically require pharmacological therapy (e.g., NSAIDs, aspiration and local steroids); quadriceps strengthening in all but very transient cases; and *cane or crutches* for joint protection in more severe problems; and they are occasionally benefited by an Ace wrap or a supportive elastic knee *sleeve* or *brace* (best avoided if there is an obvious risk of phlebitis).

The noninflammatory knee arthropathy most common in rheumatological practice is **degenerative joint disease**. This may be uni-, bi- or tri-compartmental, associated with or complicated by an inflammatory arthropathy. Degenerative joint disease of the knee is often accompanied by a periarticular problem with **medial collateral ligament strain** and **anserine bursitis** being the most common.

These mechanical disorders of the knee must be approached from the top down (Is this knee pain referred pain from an L4 discogenic radiculopathy or secondary to degenerative joint disease of the hip?) and the bottom up (Is the knee strained by compensating for a pronating foot, stiff ankle or short leg?). Knee disorders must also be approached from the standpoint of functional activity stresses such as distal fascia lata irritation of the lateral femoral condyle (**runner's knee**) or patellar tendinitis (**jumper's knee**).[75] Is the knee strained by walking with nonsupportive shoes or by bicycling? Will *orthotics* that stabilize the foot relieve knee pain? Are the *Achilles tendons or hamstrings too tight*? Is *bicycling* aggravating symptoms, and if so is it because when pedalling the knee is too flexed for patellofemoral compartment arthritis or too straight with tight hamstrings and medial tibiofemoral degenerative joint disease?[75] Is the knee pain aggravated by *over-zealous knee flexion* during a knee-chest exercise for low back pain or by attempting *deep knee bends* or *squatting* excessively as a part of a back protective regimen?

Obviously, effective management of knee disorders requires an accurate etiological diagnosis and biomechanical and functional analysis. Treatment is directed to the primary disorder (e.g., RA) when feasible, and to the local and focal painful intra- and periarticular structures (particularly the latter, as the former are only accessible by intraarticular steroid injection or arthroscopy). **Focally irritated periarticular structures** usually respond well to local ice massage, ultrasound, friction massage, and steroid injections, in about that order. Necessary measures include: *quadriceps and hamstring strengthening* (knee-extended [Fig. 78] in patellofemoral disorders to avoid patellofemoral compression, and knee in 30–60 degrees of flexion to minimize capsular strain in inflammatory and most DJD disorders [Fig. 79]); appropriate joint protection, knee support, cane, crutch, shoe-heel height, and foot

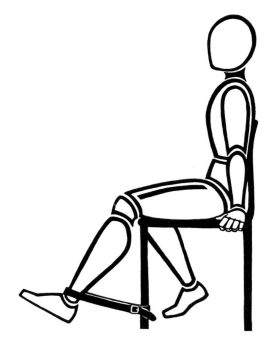

FIGURE 79. Quadriceps Strengthening.
(Seated, Belt-Resisted Isometric.)
The belt is looped around a leg of the chair for stability and the left leg attempts to overcome the belt resistance by a maximum contraction. In this illustration the knee is placed in mid-range to minimize capsular stretch pain and enhance the possibility of a forceful contraction. In patellofemoral arthroses, the knee is fully extended to minimize discomfort. In addition to the convenience of exercising in this position, the possibility that the opposite leg is incapable of offering sufficient resistance to the contraction is obviated by the use of the chair for stabilization. The contraction is held for 6 seconds and the exercise is performed once or twice daily.

stabilization; and restoration of strength to the quadriceps and hamstrings (the *goal is 95% of the strength* in the affected knee quadriceps as compared to the "good knee") before vigorous athletic activity is undertaken.[75-77]

T — Therapeutic Modalities

The inflamed knee, when either acutely or chronically involved, usually responds well to *cold packs* (20 minutes of cold pack followed by a 20- to 30-minute rest), and, when more chronic, may respond equally well or better to heat, typically as a *moist compress* for a similar period of treatment time. Cold compresses after trauma or excessive exercise and focal *ice massage for periarticular problems* are usually helpful pain control measures. These modalities are also usefully applied prior to therapeutic exercise sessions.

Ultrasound in chronic periarticular and degenerative joint disease may offer additional pain control in some cases.[11]

H — Hands-On

Hands-on therapy can be helpful in mobilizing a stiff postoperative or casted joint. *Deep friction massage over focal periarticular soft tissue irritations*, preferably after icing for analgesia, appears to ameliorate discomfort in such cases (e.g., patellar tendinitis, focal joint margin tenderness, and DJD), and gentle mobilizing maneuvers are also advocated for pain control in degenerative joint disease.[15,34]

E — Exercise

Stretching. Stretching in the face of *joint effusions* must be done cautiously *to avoid over-stretching* the joint capsule. *Serial casting or traction* can be used to treat *severe contractures* by prolonged passive stretching.

For those who would be more active physically, stretching tight quadriceps, hamstrings, or heel cords may facilitate gait and permit wearing low heels with less knee strain.

Strengthening. Strengthening for **inflammatory knee disorders** (diffuse capsular inflammations) is best done *isometrically*, with the knee held in moderate flexion in order to minimize capsular tension and pain (Fig. 79). Strengthening for **patellofemoral disorders** is least painful and most effective when done *in full extension* (Fig. 78). *Short-arc quadriceps* isotonic exercises with the leg moving from 20 to 30 degrees of flexion into full extension and then isometrically contracted for about 6 seconds can be used when an isometric contraction in either full extension or in flexion is readily performed. *Isotonic resistive exercises* to a fuller range of motion with *graduated weights* or isokinetic resistance (e.g., Cybex) can then be added to facilitate the rehabilitative program in order to achieve the maximum practical level of conditioning.[75,78,79]

R — Rest

Bedrest and occasionally casting or traction may be necessary for severe exacerbations of knee disorders. Insofar as possible, *prolonged knee flexion should be avoided at rest* in order to minimize contracture, but in an acute inflammatory disorder of anticipated short duration, sufficient knee flexion to allow for comfort is acceptable.[11]

A — ADL

Crutches or canes to avoid weight-bearing stress, *reachers* to minimize bending, proper instruction in *transfers* (bed-to-chair or chair-to-standing) to avoid strain, raised toilet seats, relatively tall and firm *chairs* and even chairs that mechanically assist in standing, and *high-low hospital beds* are all useful adjuncts to the management of knee disorders of varying severity. The use of stair railings and bathroom *grab bars* can also play a role in facilitating function and minimizing knee pain.[11]

P — Psychological Problems

Psychological needs must be addressed. The use of a cane, however necessary, must be tactfully presented, and *decorative canes*, such as "shooting sticks" (canes with fold-out seats or umbrella canes) may prove more acceptable and overcome resistance to the cane prescription.

I — Immobilization

Serial casts and resting "gutter" splints can be used for reversing contractures and maintaining extension once gained. These are primarily applied to severe chronic inflammatory knee disorders.[80] *Light-weight molded plastic orthoses* for support of a *weak, unstable knee* are available, require very careful fitting, and are not often enough effective in improving function.[81,82]

Ace wraps and *flexible elastic knee supports* give some support and comfort in a variety of knee disorders with or without instability. Various patellar apertures in elastic or rubberized splints are also available, designed to minimize patellofemoral compression and/or alter the patellofemoral interfaces, so as to minimize irritation in patellofemoral disorders. Thus far, fitting of these splints is a trial-and-error process, and care must be taken in all cases to avoid venous congestion and stasis. *Simple infrapatellar knee straps* worn during activity may help *minimize patellofemoral discomfort.*[75,83] The *athlete with major knee instability* may be rehabilitated with the use of one of several sophisticated derotation braces, such as the classic Lenox Hill derotation brace.[84]

E — Education

Apply basic principles.

S — Socioeconomic

Apply basic principles.

9. FOOT AND ANKLE DISORDERS

Knowledge of the diseases that affect the foot is crucial to our understanding of arthritic disorders and to our effectiveness in maximizing our patients' standing and ambulating abilities. Rheumatoid arthritis can affect all of the joints and adjacent tendons from the ankle distally. Rheumatoid nodules and focal bursal swelling can create painful pressure areas and a danger of ulceration infection, and rheumatoid erosions of joint surfaces or ankylosis and deformities can create painful and painfully complex ambulation problems. In patients with complicating rheumatoid vasculitis or diabetes, the propensity for neurovascular complications to affect the feet can add to the difficulties in these too-often overlooked and poorly understood anatomical regions—the feet on which our patients must rely for all of their standing and ambulatory functions.

Osteoarthritis is more selective. By and large it is relegated to the first MTP joint and the interphalangeal joint of the great toe, and occasionally to the proximal tarsal joints.

Gout notoriously affects the great toe with painful podagra and now rare painless tophi, but any part of the foot can be involved. Psoriasis in essence mimics rheumatoid arthritis, and Reiter's syndrome vascillates between resembling rheumatoid arthritis and psoriasis or both, and even gout when the foot is affected.

The Achilles heel of ankylosing spondylitis reminds us of the need to understand foot anatomy and gait kinesiology. Therefore, in order to keep in step, the clinician must be aware of the march of events that occurs during gait.[85] From *heel strike* (spondyloarthropathies, Achilles tendinitis, and bursitis) onward with ankle and hindfoot weight-bearing (*rheumatoid arthritis*, spondyloarthropathies, subtalar joint arthritis, *tarsal tunnel syndrome*, and peroneal and posterior tibial *tendinitis*), toward foot-flat (proximal tarsal and tarsometatarsal joints, *RA*, *DJD*, plantar fasciitis, calcaneal traction enthesitis, spondyloarthropathies, pronated feet, *sinus tarsi* syndrome [a very common cause of lateral foot pain with tenderness just distal to the lateral malleolus]), the problems accumulate step by step. At *foot-flat*, the plantar arch is strained during gait and particularly when standing (foot-flat—flat feet), and the metatarsophalangeal joints begin to be stressed. This MTP and plantar stress is accentuated during *heel-rise* (also a time for traction on the Achilles insertions), when weight bearing is maximal on the forefoot. At this position, especially when tight shoes are worn, *metatarsalgia* (diffusely in RA, or with hallux valgus and DJD or bunions), *sesamoiditis* (in both RA and OA, and/or post-traumatic sesamoiditis), and intermetatarsal neuralgia (*Morton's neuralgia* between the third and forth or less commonly second and third metatarsal heads) are the most common foot complaints. This is especially true in women, particularly those wearing high heels and pointed toes.[86] At *toe-off*, the first MTP and IP joints are stressed (OA) and a hyperflexed *great toe* (hallux rigidus), overlapped toes, or cocked-up toes (cavus foot, *rheumatoid arthritis* with intrinsic tightness) are pressed against a too-shallow shoe-toe box creating pain and corn and/or callus formation.[85]

This brief walk through foot mechanics and related diagnostic entities serves to illustrate the importance of etiological diagnosis, anatomic diagnosis, and functional and biomechanical diagnosis necessary to adequately treat and rehabilitate the whole foot and the whole patient in the best sense of holistic medicine.

The systemic disorders require appropriate systemic and antiinflammatory therapies, but often the latter can be minimized if the local foot problem can be relieved.[87-89] Local steroids judiciously used are a mainstay of management of focal foot problems, but whenever possible they should be used to supplement biomechanical strategies such as properly fitted supportive footwear and/or orthotics.

T — Therapeutic Modalities

Contrast baths, warm (100° F) for 5 minutes and cool (70°) for 2 minutes, repeated three to four times, ending with the cold application, are a time-honored tradition, but it is doubtful if they have any greater value than a comfortable, warm foot soak.[90] *TNS* for lower extremity neuralgia (e.g., diabetic neuropathy and reflex sympathetic dystrophy or sciatic radiculopathy) may be of value in pain control, but when wires must be extended from the belt to the ankle or foot, a sufficient nuisance can offset any but the most pronounced pain control benefit.[91]

Ultrasound and *focal ice massage* or *cold compresses* have a place in the analgesic management of foot problems, and the use of cold has the advantage of being suitable for self-administration and home therapies.[91] Particular care to avoid excessive heat or cold applications to the feet is necessary because of the commonly associated neurovascular problems.

H — Hands-On

Hands-on therapy can consist of soothing foot massage, especially on the plantar surface after prolonged walking or standing, reduction of toe subluxations, or assisted stretching (dorsiflexion) to *relieve gastroc-soleus cramps*. Pushing the foot against a foot board, dorsiflexing the foot by pulling back on the toes or getting out of bed and performing a standing heel-cord stretch can also provide relief of calf cramps (Fig. 59).

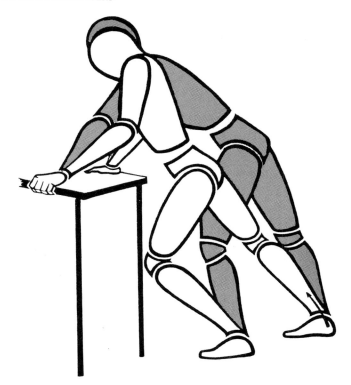

FIGURE 59 (repeated). Ankle Dorsiflexion.
(Active-Assisted Gastrocnemius-Soleus-Achilles Tendon Stretch.)

This is a vigorous stretch of the ankle plantar flexors. The patient stands before a table and extends the affected leg posteriorly. He then flexes the opposite knee while attempting to keep the foot of the affected ankle flat on the ground. By leaning toward the table, the ankle plantar flexors are stretched.

E — Exercise

Exercises for the foot and ankle are frequently mentioned but little studied.[91,92]

Stretching. Stretching of the ankle into dorsiflexion is best done with the knee bent to relieve any restriction of the gastroc-soleus-Achilles complex. By the same token, *stretching of the Achilles tendon when standing* (Fig. 59) should be performed with the forefoot slightly adducted to minimize over-stretching the calcaneus into valgus and thereby accentuating foot pronation. *Gentle stretches of the foot and ankle complex* can be made by plantar-flexing the foot and curling the toes down, then dorsiflexing the foot and flaring the toes (Fig. 80). Cupping the foot inward into supination and outward into eversion and then rotating them in clockwise and counterclockwise circles will complete a well-rounded range-of-motion exercise program for the foot. Using the toes to draw a towel across the floor is a simple mild intrinsic and extrinsic muscle conditioner for the foot (Fig. 81). *Specific contractures can be counter-stretched* to maintain mobility; e.g., early MTP dorsiflexion contractures secondary to intrinsic muscle spasm or shortening in *rheumatoid arthritis* can be treated by manual plantar flexion stretching of the MTP joints (as well as by the use of metatarsal pads in shoes with a high toe box or with sandals—see ADL).

FIGURE 80A,B. **Ankle Rotation.**

80A. The purpose of this exercise is to stretch ligaments and muscles to facilitate ankle motion. The patient is seated in a firm straight-backed chair and the feet are placed on the floor about 1 foot apart. The right heel is then moved forward a foot and a half such that the ball of the foot is about 2 to 3 inches above the ground. The heel is kept on the floor and the right foot is bent upward and inward with the great toe pointing toward the left knee. A stretch should be felt at the ankle and held for a slow count of three. 80B. With the heel on the ground, the foot is bent inward, and the right foot is bent from the ankle with the toes curling downward and forward toward the floor as far as possible. The stretch at that point is again held for a slow count of three. The heel remains on the ground and the foot is bent toward the floor; the foot is then rotated so that all the toes are pointing downward and outward and the stretch in that position is again held for a slow count of three. With the foot pointing outward, the ankle, foot and toes are then bent upward toward the knee and again the stretch is held at that point for a slow count of three. The foot is then returned to the starting position with the ball of the foot 2 to 3 inches off the floor and then relaxed. The exercise is repeated on the opposite side when indicated, and each exercise set is repeated three to five times for an optimal stretch.

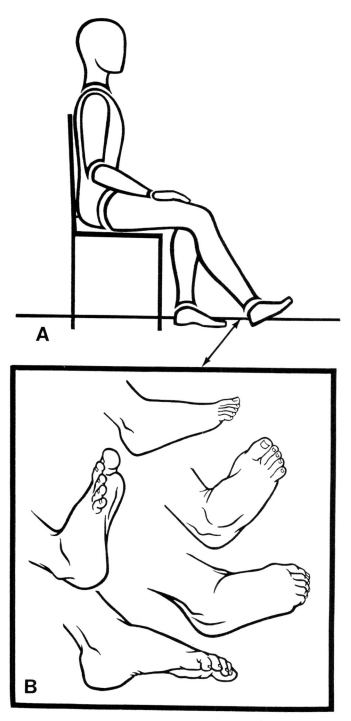

A

B

FIGURE 80A,B.   *See legend on opposite page.*

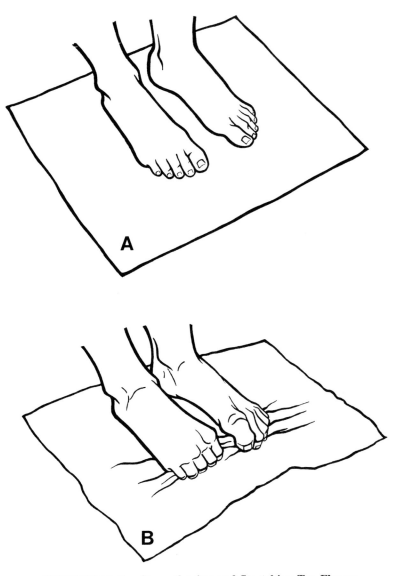

FIGURE 81A, B.   **Strengthening and Stretching Toe Flexors.**

81A. The purpose of this exercise is to stretch the muscles of the lower foot and the ligamentous support structures of the distal foot joints. The patient is seated with the feet placed comfortably side by side on a thin towel on the floor. 81B. The heels are kept flat on the towel and the towel is pulled toward the heels by a curling flexing action of the toes. This is repeated three to five times until an optimal stretch is obtained. Greater resistance can be added by placing a small weight on the towel.

Strengthening. Muscle strengthening for the foot and ankle *extrinsic muscles* (long toe extensors and flexors, peroneal muscles, and anterior and posterior tibial and gastroc-soleus muscles) are best initiated isometrically in a pain-free position. Resistance can be offered by the floor, a foot board, a door, a pillow, a bathrobe sash, a belt, a rubber hose, a heavy dental dam, a beach ball, or what-have-you.[11,92]

Isotonic exercise with low weight resistance can be added (e.g., one-pound increments) until the desired level of conditioning is achieved. It should be remembered that *weakness in myopathic muscles and neuropathic or radiculopathically denervated muscles* cannot be expected to be overcome in terms of strength greater than what is feasible in terms of the neuro- or myopathic pathology.

R — Rest

Nothing feels so good for tired and lame feet as kicking the shoes off and relaxing, preferably with the feet slightly elevated. See ADL for what to do when rest is not possible.

A — ADL

Activities of daily living of concern to the feet are walking, running, and basically anything that requires donning a shoe. *Foot protection* means protective, nonirritating footwear and/or modification of shoes by orthotics, padding or softening, and stretching points of irritation (or bandaging the foot) to relieve focal pressure and provide optimum foot support.[87–90,93] The *severely involved arthritic foot*, particularly one complicated by *impaired circulation* or *impaired innervation*, requires a *friction-free cushion-soled shoe with extra depth* in the toe box and room for a Plastizote and/or customized supportive insole. In this way, heel pressure may be relieved, excessive pronation supported, and first MTP and/or second through fifth MTP pressure relieved. The upper surface overlying the toes is ideally seamless (seams can cause focal pressures), and, for ease of adjustment, provision for multiple lace openings (greater than five pairs is preferred) is desirable. *Velcro straps and/ or elastic pretied shoelaces* can also facilitate the use of footwear in *patients with compromised hand function.*

Padding proximal to the MTP joints for *metatarsalgia* is preferably placed inside the shoe to minimize the possibility of tripping on externally placed metatarsal pads.

For the **painful ankle and hindfoot**, a *below-knee-bearing brace* (BKWB) can relieve an appreciable portion of the body weight and make otherwise too-painful ambulation possible (Fig. 82).[94,95] This brace is best combined with a cushioned (SACH) heel and a rocker sole to facilitate the transition from heel strike to toe-off during walking (Fig. 83). Recently, a leg/hind-foot orthosis to stabilize the hind-foot and ankle joints and to improve gate kinematics has been demonstrated.[92] The SACH heel and rocker sole combination may of themselves relieve sufficient ankle and/or hindfoot stress to obviate the need for bracing. This combination can also relieve mid- and forefoot strain—its main objection being a bulky shoe configuration.

For dorsiflexion weakness associated with sciatic or peripheral neuropathy, a plastic AFO (ankle foot orthosis) can relieve stumbling and fatigue from walking. An elevated heel, often further enhanced with a rocker sole, can improve the gait when there is gastroc-soleus weakness.

FIGURE 82. **Below-Knee Weight-Bearing**
(BKWB) Brace.

This brace consists of a plastic or leather molded infrapatellar upper calf cuff designed to be closely approximated to the upper one-third to one-half of the calf. A lateral and medial metal strut fixed to the shoe transmits the bulk of the body's load away from the foot and onto the lower calf. When ankle motion is painful, the ankle hinge is eliminated. Ankle motion is then simulated by a SACH heel and a rocker sole (see Fig. 83). This brace is useful in relieving stress on chronic painful refractory ankle, hindfoot and heel conditions.

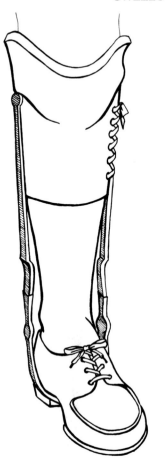

Not to be overlooked are a variety of *over-the-counter heel cushions and protective corn pads* or pressure point protectors that may prove useful for selected pressure point problems.[87,89]

The advent of stylish, light-weight *jogging shoes*, many designed to facilitate the *insertion of orthotics*, has made possible and acceptable nonmedicinal "orthopedic" shoes that can be adapted to the arthritic foot. *Severely involved and deformed feet* will require customized shoes made over casts of the foot. *Never to be forgotten* ADL items for foot problems are *canes*, *crutches*, *walkers*, and *long-handled shoehorns* for those who cannot otherwise bend over to put on their shoes.

P — Psychological Problems

Psychological problems from pain, disability and frustration with arthritic disorders are ubiquitous. The expression "my feet are killing me" may be all too real, and psychological as well as medical and/or surgical therapy has to be considered.

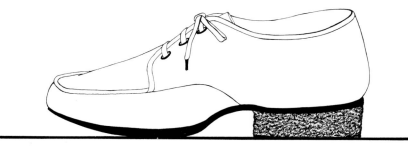

FIGURE 83. **Oxford Shoe with SACH Heel and Rocker Sole.**
The SACH, or cushion, heel absorbs the shock at heel strike and is yielding enough to give way sufficiently during the stance phase of gait to allow the foot-flat stage to be reached with only minimal ankle movement. If the cushion heel is too soft it will cause an unsteady stressful gait. The rocker sole is combined with a rigid internal shoe shank to stabilize the tarsal and MTP joints. The foot rolls over the rocker sole into the toe-off phase of gait with minimum motion of these joints or of the ankle. The cushioned heel is useful in some cases of heel pain. The rocker sole is useful in osteoarthritis of the first MTP or IP joint and when combined with a metatarsal pad may relieve the pain of severe MTP arthritis. The combination of a SACH heel and rocker sole is indicated for chronic ankle or hindfoot (proximal tarsal) arthritis. Note that a proper shoe for an arthritic foot or ankle should: (1) support the heel with a firm heel counter, (2) support the midfoot with a rigid shank, preferably with multiple lacing, and (3) allow ample room for the toes with a high toe box and a wide anterior (metatarsal area) last. Seams should not be located over dorsally protruding toe deformities.

I — Immobilization
Apply basic principles.

E — Education
Apply basic principles.

S — Socioeconomic
Apply basic principles.

GENERAL REFERENCES

Kelley WN, Harris ED Jr, Ruddy S, Sledge CB: Textbook of Rheumatology, 2nd ed. Philadelphia, W.B. Saunders, 1985.

McCarty DJ: Arthritis and Allied Conditions: A Textbook of Rheumatology. Philadelphia, Lea & Febiger, 1985.

Ehrlich GE: Rehabilitation Management of Rheumatic Conditions, 2nd ed. Baltimore, Williams & Wilkins Co., 1985.

Clark A: Rehabilitative Techniques in Rheumatology. Baltimore, Williams & Wilkins, 1987.

REFERENCES

1. Harkom TM, Lampman RM, Banwell BF, Castor CW: Therapeutic value of graded aerobic exercise training in rheumatoid arthritis. Arthritis Rheum 28:32–39, 1985.
2. Nordemar R: Physical training in rheumatoid arthritis: A controlled long-term study. II. Functional capacity and general attitudes. Scand J Rheumatol 10:25–30, 1981.
3. Swezey RL: Straight Talk on Ankylosing Spondylitis. Ankylosing Spondylitis Association, 1985.
4. Arthritis Health Professions Section of The Arthritis Foundation: Self-Help Manual For Patients With Arthritis. Atlanta, GA, The Arthritis Foundation, 1980.
5. Wolf JW Jr, Johnson RM: Cervical orthosis. In Bailey RW (ed): The Cervical Spine. Philadelphia, J.B. Lippincott Co., 1983, pp 54–61.
6. Kumar VN, Redford JB: Transcutaneous nerve stimulation in rheumatoid arthritis. Arch Phys Med Rehabil 63:595–596, 1982.
7. Melzack R, Vetere P, Finch L: Transcutaneous electrical nerve stimulation for low back pain. Phys Ther 63:489–493, 1983.
8. Thorsteinsson G, Stonnington HH, Stillwell GK, Elveback LR: Transcutaneous electrical stimulation: A double-blind trial of its efficacy for pain. Arch Phys Med Rehabil 58:8–13, 1977.
9. Paris DL, Baynes F, Gucker B: Effects of the neuroprobe in the treatment of second-degree ankle inversion sprains. Phys Ther 63:35–40, 1983.
10. Hendler N, Long DM, Wise TN: Diagnosis and Treatment of Chronic Pain. Boston, John Wright and PSG Inc., 1982, pp 77–96.
11. Swezey RL: Arthritis: Rational Therapy and Rehabilitation. Philadelphia, W.B. Saunders, 1978.
12. Swezey RL: The modern thrust of manipulation and traction therapy. Semin Arthritis Rheum 12:322–331, 1983.
13. Rath WW: Cervical traction, a clinical perspective. Orthop Rev 13:29–48, 1984.
14. Bhatt-Sanders D: Acupuncture for rheumatoid arthritis: An analysis of the literature. Semin Arthritis Rheum 14:225–231, 1985.
15. Cyriax J: Textbook of Orthopaedic Medicine, Vol. II (10th ed). London, Balliere Tindall, 1980, p 109 (Neck).
16. Cyriax J: Illustrated Manual of Orthopaedic Medicine. London; Boston: Butterworths, 1983.
17. Maigne R: Orthopedic Medicine. Springfield, IL, Charles C Thomas, 1972.
18. Tewfik ER, Christopher RP, Pinals RS, et al: Adhesive capsulitis (frozen shoulder): A new approach to its management. Arch Phys Med Rehabil 65:29–33, 1983.
19. Travell JG, Simons VG: Myofascial Pain and Dysfunction: The Trigger Point Manual. Baltimore, Williams & Wilkins, 1983.
20. Stiles EG: Safe, useful manipulative techniques. Patient Care 18:137–189, 1984.
21. Goodridge JP: Muscle energy technique: Definition, explanation, methods of procedure. J Am Osteopath Assoc 81:249–254, 1981.
22. Lorig K, Fries JF: The Arthritis Helpbook. Reading, MA, Addison Wesley, 1980, pp 67–105.
23. Arthritis Health Profession Section of The Arthritis Foundation: Self-Help Manual for Patients with Arthritis. Atlanta, GA, The Arthritis Foundation, 1980.
24. Steinbrocker O, Neustadt DH: Aspiration and Injection Therapy in Arthritis and Musculoskeletal Disorders. Hagerstown, MD, Harper & Row, 1972, p 57.
25. Olton DS, Noonberg AR: Biofeedback, Clinical Applications in Behavioral Medicine. Englewood Cliffs, NJ, Prentice-Hall, Inc., 1980, pp 202–219.
26. Seeger MW, Furst DE: Effects of splinting in the treatment of hand contractures in PSS: A controlled trial. (Submitted to Arthritis Rheum).
27. Keim HA: Fundamentals and basic principles of scoliosis. Orthop Rev 12:31–40, 1983.
28. Rothman RH, Simone FA: The Spine, Vol. I (2nd ed). Philadelphia, W.B. Saunders Co., 1982, p 339.

29. Miller JAA, Nachemson AL, Schulz AB: Effectiveness of braces in mild idiopathic scoliosis. Spine 9:632–635, 1984.
30. Calin A, Marks S: Management of ankylosing spondylitis. Bull Rheum Dis 31:35–38, 1981.
31. Rothman RH, Simone FA: The Spine, Vol. II (2nd ed). Philadelphia, W.B. Saunders Co., 1982, pp 407–413.
32. Williams PC: Low Back and Neck Pain. Springfield, Ill., Charles C Thomas, 1982, p 35.
33. Root L, Kiernan T: The Back Back Exercise Book. New York, Warner Books, Inc., pp 92–113.
34. Maitland GD: Vertebral manipulation (4th ed). London, Butterworths, 1977, p 85.
35. Krewer S: The Arthritis Exercise Book. New York, Simon & Schuster, 1981.
36. Williams PC: Low Back and Neck Pain. Springfield, Ill., Charles C Thomas, 1982, pp 20–34.
37. Jamieson RH: Exercises for the Elderly. Verplanck, New York, Emerson Books, Inc., 1982.
38. Pheasant H, Bursk A, Goldfarb J, et al: Amitriptyline and chronic low back pain: A randomized double-blind crossover study. Spine 8:552–557, 1983.
39. Levine J: Pain and analgesia: The outlook for more rational treatment. Ann Intern Med 100:269–276, 1984.
40. Ruge D, Wiltse LL: Spinal Disorders. Philadelphia, Lea & Febiger, 1977, pp 417–428.
41. Licht S: Orthotics Etcetera. New Haven, Elizabeth Licht, 1966, pp 274–302.
42. Nachemson A: Towards a better understanding of low back pain: A review of the biomechanics of the lumbar spine. Rheum Rehab 14:129–143, 1985.
43. Wiesel SW, Tsourmas N, Feffer HL, et al: A study of computer-assisted tomography. I. The incidence of positive CAT scans in an asymptomatic group of patients. Spine 9:549–551, 1984.
44. Bell G, Rothman RH, Booth RE, et al: A study of computer-assisted tomography, II. Comparison of metrizamide myelography and computer tomography in the diagnosis of herniated lumbar disc and spinal stenosis. Spine 9:552–556, 1984.
45. Irstam L: Differential diagnosis of recurrent lumbar disc herniation and postoperative deformation by myelography: An impossible task. Spine 9:759–763, 1984.
46. Cyriax J: Textbook of Orthopaedic Medicine, Vol. II (10th ed). London, Balliere Tindall, 1980, p 266 (Lumbar Back).
47. Porter PW, Hibbert C, Evans C: The natural history of root entrapment syndrome. Spine 9:418–421, 1984.
48. Quinet AJ, Hadler NM: Diagnosis and treatment of backache. Semin Arthritis Rheum 8:261–287, 1979.
49. Cailliet R: Low Back Pain Syndrome (4th ed). Philadelphia, F.A. Davis Co., 1988.
50. Deyo RA, Diehl AK, Rosenthal M: How many days of bed rest for acute low back pain? N Engl J Med 315:1064–1070, 1986.
51. Macnab I: Backache. Baltimore, Williams & Wilkins, 1977, pp 133–139.
52. McKenzie RA: The Lumbar Spine: Mechanical Diagnosis and Therapy. New Zealand, Spinal Publication, Ltd., 1981.
53. Hendler N, Long DM, Wise TN: Diagnosis and Treatment of Chronic Pain. Boston, John Wright and PSG Inc., 1982, pp 211–232.
54. Roland M, Morris R: A study of the natural history of low back pain, Part II. Spine 8:145–150, 1983.
55. Collins AJ, Notarianni LJ, Ring EFJ, Seed MP: Some observations on the pharmacology of "deep-heat," a topical rubifacient. Ann Rheum Dis 43:411–415, 1984.
56. Golden EL: A double-blind comparison of orally ingested aspirin and a topically applied salicylate cream in the relief of rheumatic pain. Curr Ther Res 24:524–529, 1978.
57. Golden EL: A Double-Blind Comparison of Orally Ingested Aspirin and a Topically Applied Salicylate Cream in the Relief of Rheumatic Pain. Current Ther Research, Vol. 24, No. 5, September, 1978, pp 524–529.
58. Russek AS: Biomechanical and physiological basis for ambulatory treatment of low back pain. Orthop Rev 5:21–31, 1976.
59. Rabinowitz JL, Feldman ES, Weinberger A, Schumacher HR: Comparative tissue absorption of oral ^{14}C-aspirin and topical triethanolamine ^{14}C-salicylate in human and canine knee joints. J Clin Pharmacol 22:42–48, 1982.
60. Judovich BD, Nobel GR: Traction therapy: A study of resistance forces. Am J Surg 93:108–114, 1957.
61. Oudenhoven RC: Gravitational lumbar traction. Arch Phys Med Rehabil 59:510–512, 1978.
62. Nosse LJ: Inverted spinal traction. Arch Phys Med Rehabil 59:367–370, 1978.

63. Lewit K, Simons DG: Myofascial pain relief by post-isometric relaxation. Arch Phys Med Rehab 65:452–456, 1984.

64. Tessman JR: My Back Doesn't Hurt Anymore. New York, Quick Fox, 1980.

65. White AH: Back School and Other Conservative Approaches To Low Back Pain. St. Louis, The C.V. Mosby Co., 1983.

66. Herron LD, Pheasant H: Bilateral laminotomy and discectomy for segmental lumbar disc disease. Spine 8:86–97, 1983.

67. Friberg O: Clinical symptoms and biomechanics of lumbar spine and hip joint in leg length inequality. Spine 9:643–651, 1983.

68. Crue BL: Chronic Pain. Jamaica, New York, Spectrum Pub., 1979.

69. Perry J: The use of external support in the treatment of low back pain. J Bone Joint Surg 52A:1140–1142, 1970.

70. Swezey RL: Pseudo-radiculopathy in subacute trochanteric bursitis of the subgluteus maximus bursa. Arch Phys Med Rehabil 57:387–390, 1976.

71. Raman D, Haslock I: Trochanteric bursitis—a frequent cause of 'hip' pain in rheumatoid arthritis. Ann Rheum Dis 41:602–603, 1982.

72. Macys JR, Bullough PG, Wilson PD Jr: Coxarthrosis: A study of the natural history based on a correlation of clinical, radiographic, and pathological findings. Semin Arthritis Rheumat 10:66–80, 1980.

73. Zizic TM, Hungerford DS, Stevens MB: Ischemic bone necrosis in systemic lupus erythematosus. Medicine 59:134–148, 1980.

74. Hungerford DS: The Hip. St. Louis, C.V. Mosby Co., 1983, pp 249–262.

75. Cailliet R: Knee Pain and Disability (2nd ed). Philadelphia, F.A. Davis Co., 1983.

76. Holden DL, Eggert AW, Butler JE: Nonoperative treatment of Grades I and II medial collateral ligament injuries to the knee. Am J Sports Med 2:340–344, 1983.

77. Helfet A: Disorders of the Knee. Philadelphia, J.B. Lippincott Co., 1974, pp 317–323.

78. Malone T, Blackburn TA, Wallace LA: Knee rehabilitation. Phys Ther 60:1602–1610, 1980.

79. Thompson NN, Gould VA, Davies BN, et al: Descriptive measures of isokinetic trunk testing. J Orthop Sports Phys Ther 7:43–49, 1985.

80. Smillie IS: Diseases of the Knee Joint. Edinburgh, Churchill Livingstone, 1974, pp 209–217.

81. Cassuan A, Wunder KE, Fultonberg DM: Orthotic management of the unstable knee. Arch Phys Med Rehabil 58:487–491, 1977.

82. Smith EM, Juvinall RC, Corell EB, Nyboer VJ: Bracing the unstable knee. Arch Phys Med Rehabil 51:22–29, 1970.

83. Levine J, Splain S: Use of the infrapatellar strap in the treatment of patellofemoral pain. Clin Orthop 139:179–181, 1979.

84. Stuller J: Bracing the unstable knee. Phys Sportsmed 13:142–156, 1985.

85. Cailliet R: Foot and Ankle Pain (2nd ed). Philadelphia, F.A. Davis, 1983.

86. Kiene RH, Johnson KA: American Academy of Orthopaedic Surgeons Symposium on the Foot and Ankle. St. Louis, C.V. Mosby Co., 1983, pp 95–101.

87. Glass ME, Karno ML, Sella EJ, Zeleznik R: An office-based orthotic system in treatment of the arthritic foot. Foot & Ankle 3:37–40, 1982.

88. Kiene RH, Johnson KA: American Academy of Orthopaedic Surgeons Symposium on the Foot and Ankle. St. Louis, C.V. Mosby Co., 1983, pp 50–80.

89. Kiene RH, Johnson KA: American Academy of Orthopaedic Surgeons Symposium on the Foot and Ankle. St. Louis, C.V. Mosby Co., 1983, pp 89–123.

90. Kottke FJ, Stillwell GK, Lehmann JF: Krusen's Handbook of Physical Medicine and Rehabilitation (3rd ed). Philadelphia, W.B. Saunders Co., 1982, p 327.

91. Bardwick PA, Swezey RL: Physical modalities for treating the foot affected by connective tissue diseases. Foot & Ankle 3:41–44, 1982.

92. Cailliet R: Foot and Ankle Pain (2nd ed). Philadelphia, F.A. Davis, 1983.

93. Wickstrom J, Williams RA: Shoe corrections and orthopaedic foot supports. Clin Orthop 70:30–42, 1970.

94. Demopoulos JT, Eschen JE: Experience with an all-plastic patellar tendon-bearing orthosis. Arch Phys Med Rehabil 58:452–456, 1977.

95. Swezey RL: Below-knee weight-bearing brace for the arthritic foot. Arch Phys Med Rehabil 56:176–179, 1978.

96. Hunt GC, Fromherz WA, Gerber L, Hurwitz SR: Hindfoot pain treated by a leg-hindfoot orthosis. Phys Ther 67:1385–1388, 1987.

97. Nutter P: Aerobic exercise in the treatment and prevention of low back pain. Spine: State of the Art Reviews 2:137–145, 1987.
98. Callahan LF, Brooks RH, Summey JA, Pincus T: Quantitative pain assessment for routine care of rheumatoid arthritis patients, using a pain scale based on activities of daily living and a visual analog pain scale. Arthritis Rheum 30:630–636, 1987.
99. Bradley LA, Young LD, Anderson KO, et al: Effects of psychological therapy on pain behavior of rheumatoid arthritis patients. Arthritis Rheum 30:1105–1114, 1987.
100. Aronoff GM, McAlary PW, Witkower A, Berdell MS: Pain treatment programs: Do they return workers to the workplace? Spine: State of the Art Reviews 2:123–136, 1987.
101. Curtis P: Spinal manipulation: Does it work? Spine: State of the Art Reviews 2:32–44, 1987.
102. Petri M, Dobrow R, Neiman R, et al: Randomized, double-blind placebo-controlled study of the treatment of the painful shoulder. Arthritis Rheum 30:1040–1045, 1987.
103. Morrey BF: The Elbow and Its Disorders. Philadelphia, W.B. Saunders, 1985.
104. Lichtman DM: The Wrist and Its Disorders. Philadelphia, W.B. Saunders, 1987.
105. Bradford DS, Lonstein JE, Moe JH, et al: Moe's Textbook of Scoliosis and Allied Spinal Deformities, 2nd ed. Philadelphia, W.B. Saunders, 1987.
106. Deyo RA, Yuh-Jane Tsui-Wu: Descriptive epidemiology of low back pain and its related medical care in the United States. Spine 12:264, 1987.
107. Breedveld FC, Algra PR, Vielvoye CJ, Cats A: Magnetic resonance imaging in the evaluation of patients with rheumatoid arthritis and subluxations of the cervical spine. Arthritis Rheum 30:624–629, 1987.
108. Deyo RA: Occupational Back Pain. Spine: State of the Art Reviews. Philadelphia, Hanley & Belfus, 1987.
109. White AH: Failed Back Surgery Syndrome. Spine: State of the Art Reviews. Philadelphia, Hanley & Belfus, 1986.
110. Linton SJ, Kamwendo K: Low back schools: A critical review. Phys Ther 67:1375–1383, 1987.
111. Deyo RA, Yuh-Jane Tsui-Wu: Functional disability due to back pain. A population-based study indicating the importance of socioeconomic factors. Arthritis Rheum 30:1247–1253, 1987.

INDEX

Pages in **boldface type** indicate complete chapters.

Pages in *italic type* indicate illustrations.